T0049390

gut

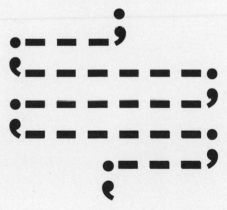

the body literacy library

gut

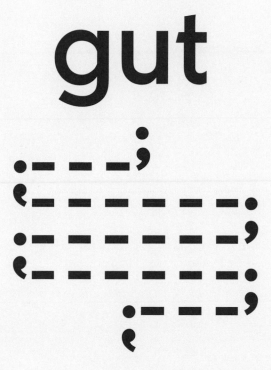

an owner's guide

Dr. Austin Chiang

the body literacy library

Body literacy is a human right. It is a means to observe,
learn, and understand ourselves—three essential steps to
enhancing our self-knowledge and self-care.

With *The Body Literacy Library,* you will learn to tune in to
every little bit of yourself. Have all your embarrassing questions
answered, and discover everything you need to know about your
body to live a happier, healthier life. This isn't just about listening
to your body but about empowering yourself with the
knowledge of what your body is telling you.

Read this book to love the skin you're in, and make informed,
positive changes to improve your health and well-being.
Starting today.

Contents

Introduction

If you think gut health is confusing, you're not alone. Contrary to popular belief, gut health is more than just intestinal health. Beyond the tube that is the esophagus, stomach, and small and large intestines, we can't forget other major organs like the liver, gallbladder, and pancreas all working collaboratively to carry out a multitude of important functions.

Many people seem to shy away from talking about gut health. The stigma around discussing butts, anuses, and poop has restricted us as a society from having important conversations about our health. And while it shouldn't be an enigma, much of gut health remains mysterious.

The onslaught of misinformation across the internet and on social media has not made gut health any easier to understand. As everyone will encounter gut health concerns at some point, many are quick to capitalize on this common ground by pushing unnecessary tests and selling supplements backed by very little evidence. Why this goes unchecked is because much of gut health is still poorly understood. Not only is the science itself still evolving, but also our understanding is constantly changing with more available evidence.

This book aims to not only clarify how your gut works but also provide guidance on what you can do to support your gut, and how we gastroenterologists treat gut health conditions when things go wrong. It's important to remember when reading this book that biology is only one determinant of gut health.

You are not entirely responsible for what is happening to your gut. Social determinants of health such as social context, access to health care and education, financial stability, and geographical location are just a few things that can affect someone's ability to coordinate their own care and follow a recommended treatment plan. Transportation, arranging childcare, or taking time off work can all impact how someone can even get to their doctor appointments. Other times, it's the availability and affordability of good food or of safe environments to remain physically active. Systemic racism and implicit bias have also impacted our health systems and how health care is practiced.

Keep in mind that doctors have based our practice of medicine on research that historically was not representative of the entire population— especially racial and ethnic minorities and sexual and gender minorities. If you fall within these groups, the greater attention today to inclusivity and health equity will hopefully help generate more evidence to better serve the gut health needs of these groups.

My aim as a gastroenterologist has always been to cut through the crap and empower everyone with evidence-based information distilled into a more digestible (pun intended) format to help you better take charge of your own gut health. But taking control of your gut health doesn't mean having to go at it alone. Let's do this together!

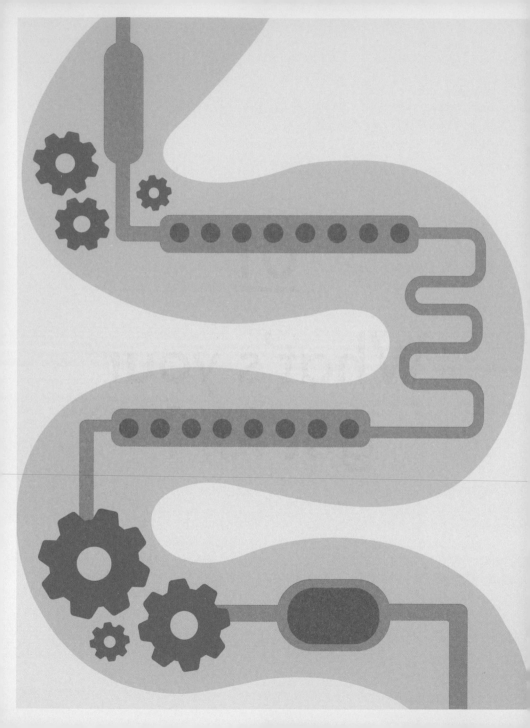

01

What's your gut for?

the clever gut

Much more than a sack of organs floating in a void, the gut is a highly sophisticated network that toils around the clock to support life.

Many people assume that the sole purpose of the gut is to extract nutrients from food while pushing out of the body whatever is left. However, the gut is much more than just a long tube connecting your mouth to your anus. Every organ of the digestive system has a specific function, and under the surface is a complex network of blood vessels, nerves, immune cells, and chemical messengers that protect you from infection, dictate when you're hungry, interact with other organs such as your brain, and more. We'll look at each organ in more detail (see pp14–17) and get into the microscopic magic behind these organs, too (see pp18–20).

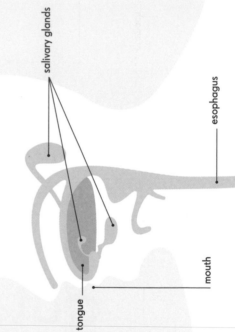

salivary glands

tongue

mouth

esophagus

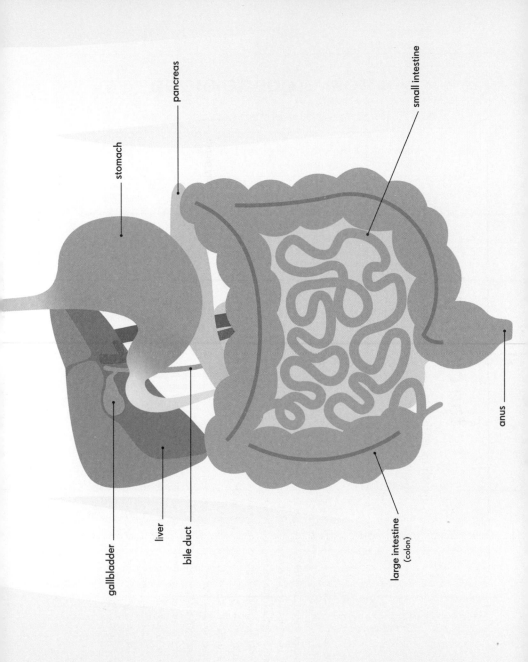

pancreas

stomach

small intestine

gallbladder

liver

bile duct

large intestine
(colon)

anus

from organ to organ

To keep the body in perfect harmony, known as homeostasis, each organ must play a specific part. Let's meet the rock-star organs in the gut ensemble!

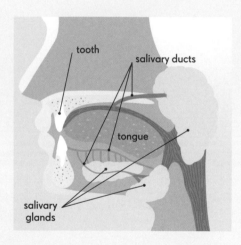

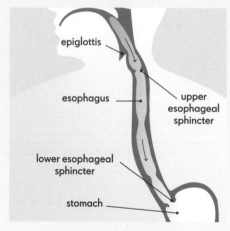

MOUTH

Digestion starts in the mouth. Your teeth cut food into small pieces. Chewing is critical to ensure food safely passes into the esophagus. In addition to this physical breakdown of food, oral enzymes found in saliva start to chemically break down complex nutrients into simpler forms that can be absorbed by the small and large intestines.

ESOPHAGUS

The esophagus is a muscular tube that actively moves food from the mouth into the stomach through a coordinated muscular movement called peristalsis. This wavelike motion propels chewed food down the esophagus to the lower esophageal sphincter, which relaxes, allowing food to enter the stomach. When you swallow, the epiglottis acts as a lid that closes over the windpipe to prevent choking.

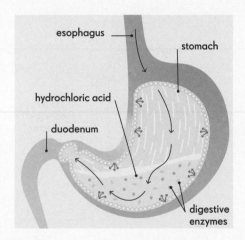

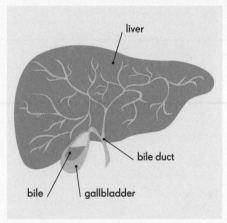

STOMACH

Your stomach is made up of multiple layers of muscle, which contract to help crush, mix, and move your food toward the small intestine. Your stomach produces hydrochloric acid and digestive enzymes, which together break down your food into a pulpy fluid called chyme. To protect itself from the gastric acid, your stomach lining secretes a layer of mucus as well as bicarbonate ions to neutralize the acid locally.

LIVER

The largest internal organ in the body, the liver performs many roles. It produces a watery green fluid called bile that helps digest fats in your food, and it makes important proteins used in blood clotting. The liver stores vitamins, minerals, and glycogen (energy) and helps clear various toxins from the body, such as alcohol and some medications.

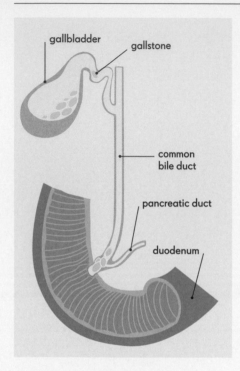

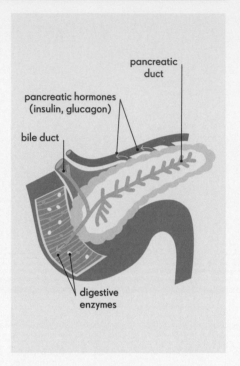

GALLBLADDER

Most of the bile produced by the liver is stored in the gallbladder; the rest goes into the small intestine. Gut hormones cause the gallbladder to contract and squeeze out bile into the duodenum to help break down fats. At times, small stones can develop and clog the outflow of bile from the gallbladder, which can lead to problems (see p151).

PANCREAS

The pancreas plays a key role in digestion and is responsible for two important functions. It makes juices containing digestive enzymes that are released into the gut to help break down proteins, carbohydrates, and fats in your food. It also makes hormones, notably insulin and glucagon, which enter the bloodstream to regulate blood sugar levels.

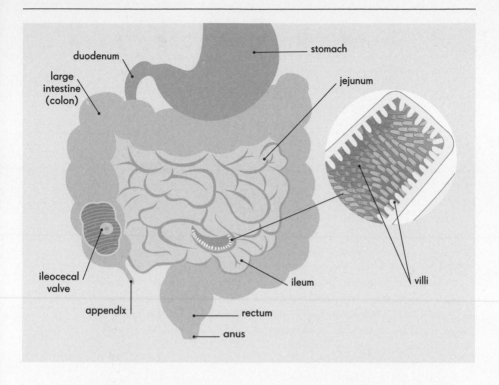

SMALL INTESTINE

The small intestine is divided into three segments: the duodenum, jejunum, and ileum, and lining the inside of each are finger like projections called villi that absorb nutrients and water from chyme. In the duodenum, digestive juices from the pancreas mix with bile from the liver to break down fats. The jejunum is comparably thicker in size and has more folds, increasing its surface area to help extract nutrients. The ileocecal valve is located at the junction of the ileum, the last part of the small intestine, and the large intestine.

LARGE INTESTINE

Shorter and wider in diameter than the small intestine, the large intestine, also called the colon, is mainly responsible for absorbing water and consolidating fecal matter. The colon plays an important role in immune function and hosts most of your gut microbiota (gut bacteria). It is also home to the appendix, a small pocket attached to the first part of the colon. The final part of your colon is the rectum, where feces are stored before being released out of the anus during a bowel movement.

under the microscope

Within each organ, there is a microscopic world of multifunctional cells that fight off invaders, make sticky secretions, and chat with other cells.

Zooming in

Every organ in the gut is made up of cells, and while some of these form the structure of the organ, others secrete important substances. Organs and cells communicate using chemical messengers like cytokines, hormones, and neurotransmitters that activate certain functions or responses in the body. Cytokines trigger immune cells to fight infection, hormones carry call-to-action messages through the blood to your organs, and neurotransmitters, released by neurons (nerve cells), activate neighboring neurons. Hormones and neurotransmitters support important functions, whether that's signaling pain and hunger, regulating blood sugar, or stimulating healing and the release of digestive juices.

The immune system

The gut is where the immune system meets the outside world in the forms of food, pollutants, toxins, and the gut's own bacteria. The gut has both physical and chemical barriers. Epithelial cells found in the gut lining act like sentinels, while the tight junctions between each of these cells form a seal. A layer of mucus covers the surface of the gut lining to keep invaders out.

The gut maintains an environment of acidity where antibacterial proteins, detergents (bile salts), and enzymes exclude unwanted bacteria. If an intruder makes it past these protective barriers, the gut has an intricate mechanism to prevent problems from escalating. In the lining of the gut, there are dendritic cells that constantly scope for "bad" bacteria, while other immune cells like macrophages remain on standby ready to fight the invaders.

In some parts of the gut, there are concentrated areas of immune cells such as Peyer's patches in the jejunum and ileum of the small intestine that trap bacteria. The immune cells T cells and B cells secrete cytokines, and immunoglobulin A (IgA), an antibody that can recognize intruders and mark them for destruction.

Cytokines signal other immune cells to fight off invaders. Sometimes (in people who are genetically susceptible) the body mistakenly identifies as harmful parts of itself, stimulating the immune cells to attack healthy cells. If these inflammatory responses remain activated over long periods of time, they can cause potentially irreversible damage to the gut. The gut microbiota is also thought to play a part in helping the immune system identify the "good" bacteria from the "bad."

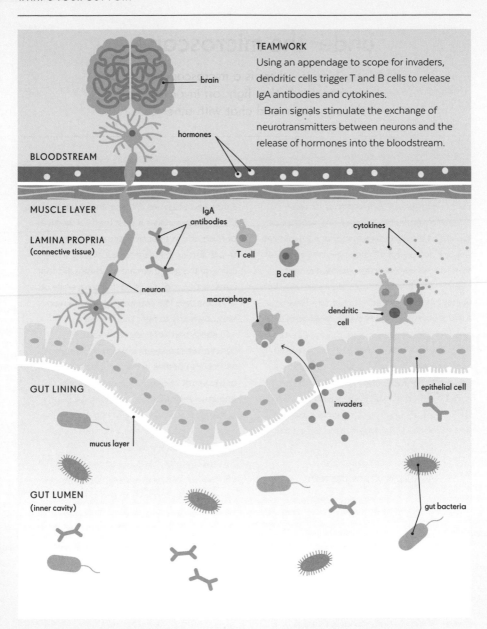

TEAMWORK

Using an appendage to scope for invaders, dendritic cells trigger T and B cells to release IgA antibodies and cytokines.

Brain signals stimulate the exchange of neurotransmitters between neurons and the release of hormones into the bloodstream.

brain

hormones

BLOODSTREAM

MUSCLE LAYER

IgA antibodies

cytokines

LAMINA PROPRIA
(connective tissue)

T cell

B cell

neuron

macrophage

dendritic cell

GUT LINING

invaders

epithelial cell

mucus layer

GUT LUMEN
(inner cavity)

gut bacteria

The nervous system

Neurotransmitters carry signals from one neuron to another or to cells in target muscles or glands. Examples of neurotransmitters are glutamate, dopamine, adrenaline, serotonin, oxytocin, GABA, histamine, and acetylcholine. They all play key roles in gut function, allowing the enteric (intestinal) nervous system to act independently of the brain, and to send and receive signals to and from the brain (see p24). These signals carry messages that help regulate functions throughout the body, including heart rate, breathing, mood, sleep, muscle movement, and many other important bodily functions.

Signals work on a lock-and-key principle—each neurotransmitter attaches to a different receptor and, when attached, triggers different types of action. There are three ways in which neurotransmitters affect neurons. Excitatory neurotransmitters stimulate an action potential, triggering a response such as muscle contraction. Inhibitory neurotransmitters slow down messaging, inducing calm and promoting sleep, while modulatory neurotransmitters influence how other neurotransmitters communicate with one another.

The endocrine system

A network of organs form the endocrine system. These organs, called glands, make hormones. Released into the blood, hormones help direct function in near and distant organs. While the hormones ghrelin and leptin communicate hunger or satiety to the brain, other hormones like gastrin tell the stomach to secrete acid in response to incoming food.

Secretin is a hormone that signals the pancreas to release pancreatic juice to help digest food and neutralize stomach acid as food enters the small intestine. Cholecystokinin is another hormone that tells the gallbladder to contract so bile is excreted into the small intestine to help digest food. Further hormones help with the speed of gut movement, regulation of blood sugar, or with cell turnover in the gut lining.

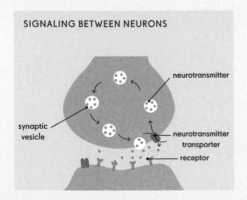

SIGNALING BETWEEN NEURONS

neurotransmitter

synaptic
vesicle

neurotransmitter
transporter

receptor

the gut microbiota

We coexist with a thriving community
of microorganisms made up from the
good, the bad, and the ugly!

It might seem strange to think that we coexist with bacteria. Yet from the moment we're born, we come into contact with them. Every day, we ingest bacteria in the foods we eat. Different foods host different bacteria. Some of these bacteria have been labeled as "good," whereas others are considered "bad." While there are some disease-causing bacteria that are unequivocally "bad," it's important to recognize that many "bad" bacteria, such as certain strains of *Escherichia coli* (E. Coli), are naturally present in our gut and cause us no harm—it's just a matter of how much of it is around. An excessive amount can be problematic.

MAPPING YOUR MICROBES
Over 100 trillion microbes live in your gut,
and most are located in the large intestine.

campylobacter

escherichia coli

enterococcus

faecalibacterium

lactobacillus

clostridium

bifidobacterium

In recent years, there has been a growing interest in how the trillions of microorganisms in our gut have the potential to help or harm our health. In addition to bacteria, there are other organisms such as fungi and viruses that may play a role. Even when focusing on bacteria, the most well-studied part of the microbiota, our understanding of how bacteria protect us from or cause certain diseases is murky at best. Scientists often use the saying, "Correlation doesn't always imply causation," meaning that while we're able to link specific bacteria to certain diseases, these *associations* do not mean that one *causes* the other, even if we have potential explanations on a microscopic level. There may be other factors to consider as well.

Each section of our gut has a unique environment (influencers include digestive juices, pH level, and oxygen concentration), and a difference in functionality, such as absorption or transportation of nutrients.

The concentration and types of bacteria also differ throughout the gut. Ultimately, what comes out the other end as feces is a collection of bacteria that scientists consider the gut microbiome, which is unique to every individual.

Dysbiosis, an imbalance in bacterial communities, within a certain part of the gut can potentially lead to disease. Multiple kinds of bacteria may be implicated in a single condition. A microbial imbalance can trigger certain processes such as inflammation, a response normally used to fight off infection. However, a prolonged or exaggerated immune response may lead to chronic inflammation and tip the body toward certain disease states, including inflammatory bowel disease (IBD), metabolic diseases (diabetes type 2, metabolic dysfunction-associated steatotic liver disease), and cancer.

When bacteria breaks down your food (or medications), metabolites are produced. These molecular compounds may interact differently with the gut lining and lead to various responses that could be good or bad for your health. One example of a metabolite is short-chain fatty acids (SCFAs) such as acetate, butyrate, and propionate. Complex carbohydrates like fiber may remain undigested until they reach the colon and are processed into SCFAs. These SCFAs may play a role in various diseases by interacting with receptors (binding proteins in cells) within the gut lining, leading to hormonal and immune responses. How we modify the bacteria to make more or less of these by-products has

• MICROBIOTA VS. MICROBIOME •

The terms "microbiota" and "microbiome" are often used interchangeably, but there is a difference. Microbiota describes the microorganisms (bacteria, viruses, and fungi) that live in the gut, whereas microbiome refers to both the microorganisms and their genetic material.

become a growing area of interest for research. So where do we go from here? Many scientists are looking for ways to alter the gut microbiome to our benefit, to reduce disease and help us lead longer, healthier lives. Much research has been focused on adding beneficial prebiotics and probiotics to the foods we eat. Prebiotics, a form of dietary fiber, promote the growth of some types of bacteria. Probiotics are specific strains of bacteria consumed in certain supplements and foods, like yogurt. Some medications play a role in changing the composition of the gut microbiota. Antibiotics can alter gut microbiota by destroying certain kinds of bacteria, including potentially helpful ones. This is why antibiotics should not be used to treat illnesses that will get better by themselves, such as a cold, but instead should be reserved for serious infections. Although

what we can do to tip the balance of bacteria in our favor isn't well understood, many gastroenterologists recommend eating a varied diet to make sure that the balance isn't tipped in one particular direction.

There are well-established methods of taking an individual's entire microbiome and transplanting it into someone else in the form of a fecal microbiota transplant (FMT). This procedure is carried out in a hospital.

Some diarrheal conditions like *Clostridioides difficile* infection can recur. However, these recurrences can be prevented by taking poop from a healthy donor and giving it to someone else (sometimes in capsules ingested by mouth or delivered into the rectum). There are ongoing studies on how this therapy can help with other conditions, including obesity and autoimmune disorders.

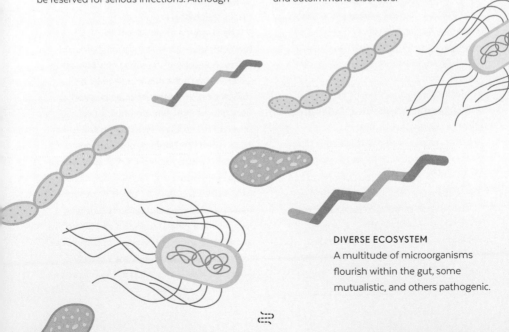

DIVERSE ECOSYSTEM
A multitude of microorganisms flourish within the gut, some mutualistic, and others pathogenic.

two-way communication

You can't hear the conversations, but your gut is in
constant dialogue with other organs, sending and
receiving call-to-action messages.

The gut does not operate in isolation but rather
is intimately connected to other parts of the
body. The gut is thought to communicate with
other organs, and the gut microbiota is believed
to be the driver of this internal dialogue.

The gut-brain axis

The gut-brain axis describes signaling
between the gut and the central nervous
system. This relationship is not one-sided.
Communication between the gut and the brain
can occur in both directions. Part of what makes
this interaction possible is that the gut has an
entire nervous system of its own. Often referred
to as the "second brain," the enteric (intestinal)
nervous system includes neural connections to
the spinal cord and the brain. At baseline, the
gut can move on its own, thanks to this second
brain. But gut movement can also be affected
by external signals from the brain and by the
gut microbiota.

As much as the brain's emotional state
can impact the gut, the gut in turn can send
signals back to the brain. When discussing the
gut-brain axis, many are referring specifically to
the microbiota-gut-brain axis. Some of the gut
microbiota signals are local to the intestine,
but others travel to the brain, via the vagus
nerve and spinal cord, and are associated
with certain neurological or psychological
conditions. We know that when processing
food, gut bacteria produce certain by-products
that can trigger immune, hormonal, or neural
responses. Also, in response to certain foods,
the gut microbiota may alter gut permeability,
allowing unwanted substances to enter the
bloodstream, thereby affecting the nervous
system. The low-grade inflammation that
results from the presence of these intruders
may have a role in certain neurological
diseases, but this is still not well understood.
To date, it's unclear how much the gut
microbiota is related to neurological disorders
like Parkinson's disease, and Alzheimer's
disease, or psychiatric conditions such as
depression. Keep in mind that while the gut
microbiota may be different in people with a
certain disease, scientists are not able to say
for sure that gut bacteria is the direct cause
of the disease.

The most cited disorder of the gut-brain
axis is irritable bowel syndrome (IBS). IBS is
characterized by recurring abdominal pain
with altered bowel habits. Not only do
conditions like anxiety and depression put
people at higher risk of developing IBS, but
those with IBS also have a higher risk of

developing anxiety and depression. When looking at IBS from a brain-to-gut perspective, there is evidence that the brain exerts an effect on both the movement and sensitivity of the gut.

The exact relationship between the gut and the brain is difficult to study and define as there are so many types of gut disorders, variable compositions of gut microbiota, and differences in environment and diet. Disorders of the gut often come in different forms (even IBS has various subtypes), and gut microbiota can vary greatly between two people with the same condition and can be influenced by where they live and what they eat, too. Similarly, brain activity is not always constant: sleep, stress, and other factors can alter brain function.

Without the ability to target the gut-brain axis in its entirety, treatments for disorders like IBS are limited. Some focus on symptoms (brain), while others try to focus on function (gut). One of the most recommended treatments to reduce IBS symptoms, such as excess gas and bloating, is a low-FODMAP diet, which excludes a group of carbohydrates known as fermentable oligosaccharides, disaccharides, monosaccharides, and polyols found in certain fruits and vegetables such as apples and onions. The effects of this diet on the gut microbiota and how it may change over time are not well understood. Likewise, medications aimed at altering gut function (such as those prescribed for constipation-predominant IBS) may help alleviate symptoms but do not serve to alter the gut microbiota or the behavioral inputs relevant to this condition.

INTERNAL DIALOGUE

The gut and brain exchange information bidirectionally using hormones that travel through the bloodstream and neurotransmitters that communicate through the nervous system, notably via the vagus nerve, the main highway for signals to travel between the brain and gut.

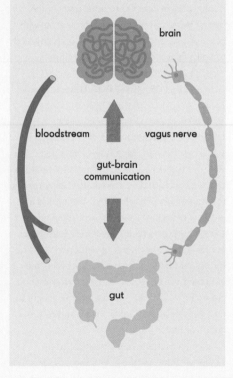

brain

bloodstream

vagus nerve

gut-brain communication

gut

The gut-endocrine axis

Glands make hormones, including those that help regulate appetite. This is a major part of how the gut interacts with the endocrine system. Gut hormones ghrelin and leptin message your brain when you are hungry or full. When these signals don't function properly, certain conditions such as obesity and metabolic diseases can result.

With the advent of weight loss surgery (also called bariatric surgery), researchers have gained a better understanding of hunger and fullness signals by looking at how weight loss patients respond following the surgical removal of certain segments of their gut. For example, a gut hormone found to suppress appetite and provide a sense of fullness is glucagon-like peptide-1 (GLP-1). In recent years, this hormone has become a major focus for multiple diabetes and weight loss medications (GLP-1 agonists). Several of these drugs, such as semaglutide, are now FDA-approved and are beginning to transform the medical approach to weight loss for those with morbid obesity.

Some believe the gut microbiome to be the body's largest endocrine organ, home to various gut hormones. How the gut microbiota interacts with these specific gut hormones is an area of much research. Scientists have been excited by the potential to activate gut bacteria in a way that may help promote weight loss, although, to date, no specific prebiotic or probiotic remedy, supplement, or other product has been found to target the gut-endocrine-microbiota axis effectively and reliably.

Besides appetite, another aspect of the gut-endocrine axis is the ability of the gut to know what foods are being eaten and what digestive enzymes are needed to break down carbohydrates, proteins, and fats. To help in the digestion of these macronutrients, hormones trigger the secretion of certain digestive juices, like bile from the gallbladder.

Some believe the gut microbiome to be the body's largest endocrine organ.

The gut-skin axis

The gut and skin have some similar characteristics. They are teeming with bacteria and both act as the body's first line of defense to the outside world, and they share some protective mechanisms, too. Both the gut and skin act as barriers against outside pathogens. When scientists talk about the gut-skin axis, some are referring to the interaction between the gut microbiota and the skin.

One way to think about the gut-skin axis is to consider the many skin findings (clinical observations) linked to various gut health conditions. For example, Leser-Trelat sign describes pigmented skin lesions that may indicate possible cancer in the abdomen. Jaundice is another example where the yellowing of the skin is the result of a buildup of bile. Sometimes one gut disease can cause multiple different skin findings that are not exclusive to that one condition. In cirrhosis, two skin findings include redness in the palms (known as palmar erythema) and Terry's nails (discoloration of the nail bed), both of which are not specific to cirrhosis alone.

The relationship between food and skin is also a hot topic. Some examples of this relationship are clearer than others. Patients with celiac disease may develop dermatitis herpetiformis, an itchy, blistering skin condition affecting about 10 percent of patients. Fortunately, this skin condition will often clear up after a few weeks if the patients adopt a gluten-free diet. (Gluten is a protein that causes the immune system in a celiac to damage the gut lining.) The relationship between the gut microbiota and acne is less clear. There are many triggers and causes of acne, and associations have been made when comparing the microbiota of patients with acne versus those without. However, the mechanism of the relationship between the gut and acne remains unclear and as a result, there is no targeted, one-size-fits-all diet to treat acne.

the history of gut medicine

Our understanding of gut health has evolved hugely,
from testing early surgical devices on sword swallowers
to using robotic arms and tools in theater.

16th to 18th centuries

Ancient Greece

One of the first mentions of gut health came
from the ancient Greek physician Hippocrates
(460–377 BCE) who noted, "All diseases begin
in the gut." Although not entirely accurate,
this early theory is nonetheless insightful.
Hippocrates also coined one of the first
documented references to digestive health
by naming digestion "pepsis." This word can
be found today in conditions referring to the
stomach, such as dyspepsia. Centuries later,
fellow Greek physician Galen (130–200 CE)
theorized that the stomach minced food,
the intestines decomposed it, and the
blood vessels transported nutrients to the
liver through blood vessels. His theory
remained accepted until the 17th century.

Belgium-born anatomist and physician
Andreas Vesalius (1514–1564) accurately
described gastrointestinal anatomy based
on his findings from conducting human
autopsies. The following century, Dutch
physician Franciscus Sylvius (1614–1672)
was the first to identify the roles of saliva
secretions and the chemical actions of stomach
acid and alkaline bile in the small intestine in
the digestive process. The first reference to
gut microbiota can be traced back to 1683
when Dutch microbiologist and microscope
master Antoine van Leeuwenhoek described
differences in his oral and fecal bacteria.

Early 20th century

In the early 20th century, our understanding of digestive chemistry accelerated. In 1902, British physiologists Sir William Bayliss (1860–1924) and Ernest Starling (1866–1927) first identified the hormone secretin, a gut hormone that aids digestion by stimulating the liver and pancreas. Russian physiologist Ivan Pavlov (1849–1936; famous for Pavlov's dog experiments) was awarded the Nobel Prize in 1904 for first describing brain-gut interactions. Pavlov discovered that signals delivered via the vagus nerve triggered stomach secretions. A year later, British physiologist John Edkins (1863–1940) identified gastrin, a gut hormone that stimulates acid secretion in the stomach. By 1916, Leon Popielski (1866–1920), a Polish doctor, learned how histamine stimulates stomach acid secretion. (In 1988, Sir James W. Black [1924–2010] a British physician and pharmacologist, received a Nobel Prize for developing the first histamine receptor blocker medication to control stomach acid production.)

Insulin, the sugar-regulating hormone made by the pancreas, was first discovered in 1921 by Canadian surgeon Sir Frederick Banting (1891–1941) and scientist J. J. R. Macleod (1876–1935). In 1923, the two were awarded the Nobel Prize, and the first shipment of mass-produced insulin was made the same month.

Breakthroughs made in other scientific fields, such as the discovery of penicillin in 1928 by bacteriologist Sir Alexander Fleming (1881–1955), changed our understanding of digestive disease.

18th to 19th centuries

The first procedures to treat gastrointestinal conditions were documented in the 18th to 19th centuries. In 1735, French surgeon Claudius Amyand (1660–1740) removed a perforated appendix (an inflamed appendix that had burst) in an 11-year-old boy, making it the first documented appendectomy. In 1868, German surgeon Adolph Kussmaul (1822–1902) fashioned the first gastroscope to investigate the upper gastrointestinal tract using a 18.5 in (47 cm) long rigid metal tube and mirror lit by a gas lamp. Using this device, he attempted to explore the esophagus and stomach of professional sword swallowers at a meeting attended by fellow physicians. (It wasn't until 1932 that a degree of flexibility into the scope was introduced by German gastroenterologist Rudolph Schindler [1888–1968], now considered the "father of gastroscopy.")

Mid-20th century

Major progress was made in procedural interventions in the mid-20th century. In a publication from 1935, American surgeon Allen Whipple (1881–1963) first described the Whipple procedure, a surgery now mostly used in the treatment of pancreatic cancer. Regarded as the "father of modern transplantation," American surgeon Thomas Starzl (1926–2017) performed the world's first liver transplant in 1963. Around this time, other significant improvements were made to the endoscope, including a fully flexible fiber-optic endoscope developed by South African gastroenterologist Basil Hirschowitz (1925–2013). By 1969, the first fiber-optic colonoscope long enough to examine the entire colon was developed.

Late 20th century

In the late 20th century, rapid developments were made to help make procedural interventions safer. Before the hepatitis C virus was discovered in 1992, patients undergoing surgery would receive transfusions using blood that had not been screened for this virus. Direct-acting antiviral medications introduced 20 years later would improve hepatitis C cure rates to nearly 100 percent. Surgical procedures also became less invasive with the first laparoscopic cholecystectomy (gallbladder removal) in 1986, which became a flagship procedure for laparoscopic surgery. Later in 1999, this "keyhole" approach to surgery was applied to the first laparoscopic sleeve gastrectomy, now the most performed weight loss surgery.

In 1985, US President Ronald Reagan underwent a colonoscopy that revealed a tumor. He later underwent surgery to have a segment of his colon removed. By the mid-1990s, the first colorectal cancer screening recommendations were set. Newer less-invasive treatment methods also emerged in the 1990s, where early tumors could be removed by using an endoscope to avoid surgical removal of entire sections of the gut.

Early 21st century

In 2005, Australian physicians Barry Marshall (1951-) and Robin Warren (1937-) were awarded the Nobel Prize for their discovery in 1979 of *Helicobacter pylori*, a bacteria linked to stomach inflammation, ulcers, and cancer.

Following the death of her husband at age 42 from colon cancer, American journalist Katie Couric had a colonoscopy live on television in March 2000 in the hope of reducing stigma and to raise awareness of gut health. The ability to examine the small intestine and colon improved further with the introduction of capsule endoscopy in the early 2000s, allowing doctors to examine the gut without a procedure. This technology was later applied in the UK for colorectal cancer screening during the COVID-19 pandemic.

In 2008, a fecal microbiota transplant was first used to treat recurrent *Clostridioides difficile* infection, reintroducing an ancient treatment method to remedy a specific condition of the gut. In 2021, the first artificial intelligence-powered device to help doctors identify polyps during a colonoscopy was approved by the FDA, heralding a new era of technology in gastroenterology. The same year, the recommended colorectal cancer screening age was lowered from 50 to 45 for average-risk individuals in the US.

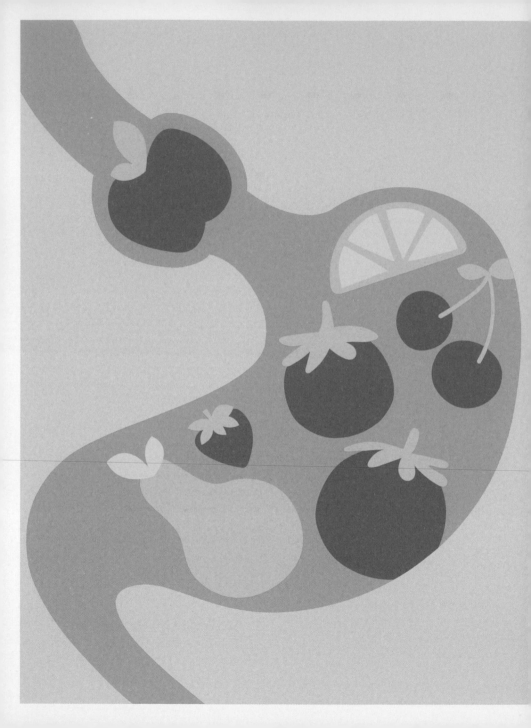

02

Digestion and Nutrition

how digestion works

Digestion involves both the mechanical and chemical breakdown
of food, starting from the mouth and ending at the anus.

The goal of digestion is to break down the foods that we consume so that our body can extract the nutrients to provide energy and other benefits to help us survive and thrive. Some may argue that digestion starts with the brain. When you see or smell food, the brain signals the salivary glands to produce saliva. When food enters your mouth, chewing mechanically breaks down food into smaller pieces, which allows enzymes and other digestive juices to chemically digest your food. One of the key enzymes released by the salivary glands is amylase, which helps break down carbohydrates like complex starches into simpler sugars.

After food is chewed, the bolus (ball of partially digested food) is swallowed and swept backward into your pharynx by the tongue. When food is actively swallowed, the epiglottis (a flap of tissue) closes over your trachea (windpipe) so that food is directed into the esophagus rather than your lungs. Using wavelike contractions called peristalsis, the muscles of the esophagus push the bolus down into your stomach where it gets churned and mixed with gastric juices to create chyme, a semiliquid mixture.

Chemical digestion also occurs in the stomach as its lining makes hydrochloric acid to create an acidic environment to denature proteins, helping to unfold their molecular structure. Enzymes like pepsin break down proteins further into their individual components: amino acids.

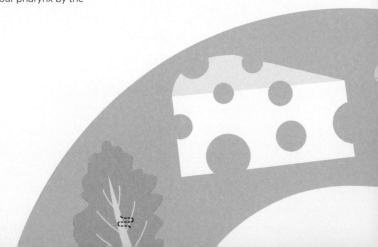

The chyme then enters your small intestine, where most of the absorption and digestion occurs. Peristalsis continues to propel the partially digested food forward through the intestines. To increase the surface area of the small intestine to absorb more nutrients, the wall of the small intestine has fingerlike projections called villi, and each villi contains microvilli. In the small intestine, food mixes with other digestive juices like bile and pancreatic juices that empty into the first portion of the small intestine, the duodenum.

Bile, which is made by the liver, can break down triglycerides (dietary fats) into smaller droplets, allowing other enzymes like lipase to further process the fats. Lipase, which is made by the pancreas, breaks down fats into fatty acids and glycerol. Pancreatic juices not only contain lipase but also trypsin, another enzyme that breaks down protein, and more amylase.

From the small intestine, the chyme continues its journey moving into your large intestine (colon) where the primary function is absorbing water and minerals. This is where poop starts to become more solid. The colon is also home to most of your gut microbes, the bacteria that ferments undigested foods and produces gases. The leftover undigested waste and bacteria then accumulate in the rectum (the last segment of the colon), which stretches the walls of the intestine, creating the urge to poop.

Other ways of feeding and pooing

When digestion is impaired, other methods of feeding are needed to move food past the diseased area of the gut. For patients who are unconscious or unable to chew, a feeding tube may need to be inserted into their stomach to deliver liquid nutrition. For a more permanent solution or for patients with an obstructing esophageal mass, food may need to be delivered directly into the stomach through a percutaneous gastrostomy (PEG) tube that is inserted through the skin. If digestion or emptying of the stomach is impaired (as in the case of gastroparesis, see p128, or an obstructing tumor), tube insertion further downstream with a percutaneous jejunostomy (PEJ) may be required.

When patients are unable to tolerate any sort of feeding via the gut, parenteral nutrition (or nutrition delivered intravenously) may be required.

When segments of the intestines are removed due to diseases like ulcerative colitis, a temporary or permanent outlet may be surgically created for waste to be emptied out of the gut through the skin. These ostomies allow waste to empty from either the small intestine or the large intestine.

Other surgical alterations in anatomy can create nutritional and digestive challenges. For patients who have undergone gastric bypass for weight loss, some of this is intentional. However, reduced nutrient absorption can result because of bypassing certain segments of the gut.

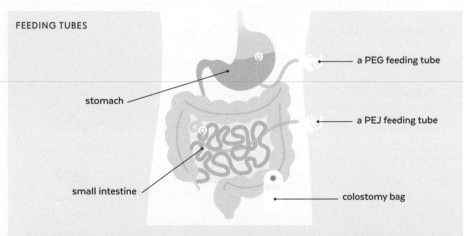

FEEDING TUBES

a PEG feeding tube

stomach

a PEJ feeding tube

small intestine

colostomy bag

When unable to feed by mouth, a tube can be inserted either into the stomach or small intestine to directly deliver nutrition into the gut. Depending on the underlying cause, these tubes can remain in place indefinitely.

foreign body ingestions

Each year, there are tens of thousands of cases of
foreign body ingestion resulting in visits to the hospital.

While some people accidentally swallow objects, others may do so due to underlying psychiatric disorders. Depending on the size, some of these items can become lodged within the esophagus, while others get lodged further downstream in the intestine. The longer something is stuck, the greater the risk of an ulcer or perforation of the gut wall, which could prove deadly. Smaller objects may pass through the gut safely, eventually being released into the toilet.

Common foreign body ingestions in adults	Common foreign body ingestions in children
• Fish and chicken bones	• Coins
• Dentures	• Plastic toys
• Silverware	• Marbles
• Toothbrushes	• Crayons
• Illicit drugs	• Nails, pins
• Narcotic packets	• Button batteries
	• Magnets
	• Caustic substances

What to do?

Most items swallowed will pass through the gut, but 10-20 percent will require medical intervention. As a rule of thumb, small round objects less than the size of a penny can safely pass through the gut and not get held up along the way by any sphincters. The major exceptions are a disc or button battery, as it can burn through the gut wall, and small magnets, as they can couple between loops of the bowel. Anything long and/or sharp that can't make the natural turns in the intestine may have to be retrieved using endoscopic tools. In severe cases, an endoscopy may not be enough, and surgery may be required to remove the object.

Narcotic packets (typically ingested by drug smugglers) need to be removed surgically because endoscopic removal may risk damaging the drug packets and causing an overdose. Caustic agents include alkali or acidic agents, often in household cleaning agents. These agents can damage and melt away layers of the gut wall. If a hole has burned through the esophagus or stomach, surgery may be required to remove the damaged part. Inducing vomiting is not a good idea as it may increase the risk of a perforation if the wall is already damaged. Long term, there can be consequences of scarring and strictures (narrowing) that happen over the following weeks to years, as well as an increased risk of cancer.

• CHOKING VERSUS ESOPHAGEAL FOOD IMPACTION •

Choking is when your airway gets blocked. Thanks to the epiglottis, food is directed down your esophagus rather than your windpipe. But when food goes down the wrong tube into the airway, choking can happen. This can be immediately life threatening as air cannot move into your lungs to breathe. That's why abdominal thrusts are performed to force the object out of the airway.

Food impaction is when something gets stuck in the esophagus. Sometimes the object is too big. Other times there is an underlying condition in the esophagus such as tumors, or other muscle movement disorders that prevent food from going down. Aside from treating the underlying cause, the food or object needs to be removed to clear the passage.

eating disorders

Eating disorders are mental illnesses with
associated behaviors that often involve the gut.

Eating disorders affect at least 9 percent of people worldwide. Because patients with these disorders are often not able or willing to disclose their difficulties in maintaining a healthy weight, diagnosis can sometimes be missed or delayed. These disorders likely stem from multiple causes, where body dissatisfaction, exposure to negative comments, a perceived lack of control, underlying genetic contributions, and other neurobiological factors result in disordered eating behavior.

Evaluation of these conditions not only involves objective measurement of weight and caloric intake, and assessment of nutrient levels, but also looking for physical signs of malnutrition and purging behaviors. This may include cardiac arrhythmias, menstrual abnormalities, skin changes like brittle hair and nails or lanugo (fine, soft body hair because of malnutrition), knuckle scraping from self-purging behaviors, and dental erosion from repeated vomiting. Common gastrointestinal symptoms with eating disorders include constipation (because of nutritional deficiencies and low volume intake), nausea, vomiting, bloating, and abdominal pain. In patients with frequent vomiting, GERD (gastroesophageal reflux disease, see p98), Barrett's esophagus (see p98), and Mallory-Weiss tears (see p129) can be found.

Treating eating disorders often requires a multifaceted approach with various medical specialists to address not only the underlying mental illness but also any nutritional issues and other medical complications. In addition to psychotherapy and psychiatric medications, weight management under the guidance of a dietitian (and close observation in the hospital) may be required in severely malnourished patients to prevent dangerous consequences from refeeding syndrome, including seizures, heart failure, and death. To follow are eating disorders I often encounter in clinic.

Anorexia nervosa is a disorder of significantly low weight, fear of gaining weight, and a disturbance in body image. There are two subtypes: restrictive type (dieting, fasting, exercising), and binge eating/purging type.

Bulimia nervosa is a disorder of recurrent binge eating behavior with inappropriate purging behaviors to compensate for weight gain. These behaviors may include self-induced vomiting, laxative, enema, and diuretic use, or stimulant abuse. Nonpurging behaviors to control weight include excessive physical activity, fasting or restricting intake, or withholding insulin doses in patients with diabetes. Unlike those with anorexia nervosa, patients with bulimia nervosa may have a normal weight on physical examination. However, maintaining the semblance of normal weight is often a result of poor self-image and an excessive preoccupation with calorie counting.

Binge eating disorder is defined by weekly binge episodes over a period of at least three months. Although binge eating disorder often results in overweight, weight is not a part of the criteria for this diagnosis. Some associated symptoms include eating regardless of hunger or satiety and negative feelings after binge episodes. Sometimes binge eating disorder does not develop until after patients gain excess weight.

Avoidant restrictive food intake disorder (ARFID) is a disorder that results in significant weight loss caused by the fear of consuming certain foods due to texture, smell, appearance, or fear of nausea, constipation, or other allergic reaction. Unlike anorexia nervosa or bulimia nervosa, patients with ARFID do not have excessive concerns about their body weight or image.

Pica is a disorder where nonfood substances, such as chalk, laundry powder, soil, or paint chips, are ingested. While pica can also describe patients who ingest ice, a possible symptom of anemia, this does not inherently present a toxic health risk the way paint chips might. Consumption of some of these items may also be of cultural significance, in which case it is not considered a disorder.

Rumination disorder is when food is automatically regurgitated and swallowed again to self-soothe and can occur in both children and adults. To fulfill the criteria, this behavior must occur for more than a month and not be linked to an underlying gastrointestinal (GI) condition.

Treating eating disorders often requires a multifaceted approach.

overweight and obesity

These medical conditions are characterized
by an excess accumulation of body fat.

Having excess body fat may carry a greater risk of health consequences, including heart disease and various cancers. How overweight and obesity are categorically defined is often based on a measurement called body mass index, or BMI, which is measured by mass (kg or lbs) divided by height (ft or m) squared. BMI has been widely criticized as an inaccurate way to assess weight status, as greater mass does not always represent greater amounts of fat. For example, bodybuilders often have a high BMI due to greater muscle mass and some people with high BMI may be objectively healthier in other ways than someone who simply falls into the "normal" BMI category.

While overweight and obesity are a result of consuming more calories than are spent, managing weight is very complex. Not only are there variations in the biology of our human bodies between individuals, but there are differences in environment, lifestyle, and behavioral factors, too. For example, hormonal imbalances affecting appetite may differ from one person to the next, and how many calories are retained in response may also differ.

External factors like inconsistent work schedules, sedentary lifestyle, and limited access to healthy food options may increase the risk of gaining weight. By way of example, someone genetically predisposed to gaining weight who lives in an obesogenic (producing obesity) environment, engages in limited physical activity, and has an excess of food energy may experience more easily an accumulation of fat.

Overweight and obesity are public health concerns, with 41.9 percent of US adults categorized as obese and 30.7 percent classed as overweight, according to the National Health and Nutrition Examination Survey (NHANES). Health professionals are often not only concerned about the impact excess body fat has on overall health but also the economic burden these conditions and their complications may cause for the greater society.

Discussing overweight and obesity is a sensitive subject. The topic of weight is heavily stigmatized, making it more difficult for patients to seek and execute treatment plans. The "body positivity" movement was developed to challenge societal beauty standards and advocate for inclusivity and acceptance of diverse body shapes and sizes. While body positivity should be embraced to reduce stigma, it is important that conversations around weight and health are had but not forced upon the individual nor encouraged for cosmetic purposes. Various medical organizations have also outlined best practices to help reduce stigma, create a comfortable environment, and ensure appropriate language is used when discussing weight. Ultimately, the decision to lose weight is a personal one. For those seeking to lose weight, the goal is not necessarily to achieve a "normal" body weight but rather to lose enough weight to reduce the risk of other health problems. Moreover, the best treatment is one that can be sustained long term.

Because of its many causes and influences, treatment for overweight and obesity is often multifaceted. Dietary adjustments and lifestyle changes are the cornerstone of treatment, with many commercial weight loss programs helping patients limit caloric intake. Addressing other associated conditions such as diabetes, sleep apnea, psychiatric disorders, and more, together with social determinants, including work patterns, social support, and environmental concerns like safe neighborhoods

to remain physically active and food deserts, are equally important in helping individuals lose weight effectively.

Today, there are oral and injectable weight loss medications available to help achieve weight loss. Surgical weight loss procedures include the Roux-en-Y gastric bypass (where the intestines are rerouted to allow food to skip the stomach and part of the small intestine) or laparoscopic sleeve gastrectomy (where part of the stomach is removed to limited how much food the stomach can hold). Endoscopic procedures through the mouth are also becoming increasingly popular, including intragastric balloons (balloons that temporarily occupy space in the stomach) and the endoscopic sleeve gastroplasty (where the stomach is sewn down to a smaller size to help limit intake).

CUT IN TWO

To limit the food a morbidly obese individual can eat at one time, an operation is performed to reduce the size of the stomach and the hunger hormones produced. A sleeve gastrectomy (bariatric surgery) divides the stomach in two, leaving a narrow "sleevelike" tube.

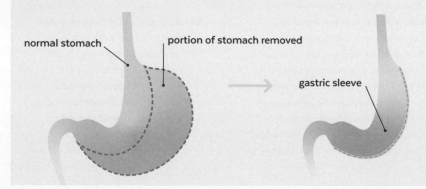

normal stomach

portion of stomach removed

gastric sleeve

food allergies and intolerances

Reactions that are immune-mediated are allergies,
whereas non-immune-mediated reactions are intolerances.

Reactions to food are often confusing because not all are easily diagnosed, there may be variability in how different people experience the same reaction, and the mechanisms are sometimes not well understood. Symptoms experienced are neither more nor less comfortable with one or the other reaction, and the treatment is quite different.

Between 2007 and 2011, rates of food allergies increased by 50 percent among children in the US, and in the UK, overall admissions to hospital for food-related anaphylaxis increased threefold between 1998 and 2018. There are theories as to why this may be, but they are largely inconclusive. However, many scientists agree that lifestyle and environmental changes and their impact on the microbiome have a significant role.

Food allergies reportedly affect about 8 percent of children and between 2 and 10 percent of all adults in the US. The UK has some of the highest prevalence rates of allergic conditions in the world, with over 20 percent of the population affected by one or more allergic disorders. The most common allergens among young children include milk, eggs, peanuts, tree nuts, and wheat. Children often outgrow most of these allergies, with peanuts and tree nuts being the exception. It is unclear why this happens, but theories include changes in the microbiome, maturing of the immune system, and changes in the gut lining with age.

Many adults develop allergies to foods later in life, with shellfish and raw fruit being the most common. Some scientists think this delayed response may be because food allergens were not introduced in childhood thereby exposing the immune system at an early age. Evidence suggests that a raw fruit allergy may be related to having a pollen allergy—postharvest, pollen can linger on raw fruit. Considering how many different foods, bacteria, and foreign things travel through our

• TOP ALLERGENS •

According to the FDA, the nine major food allergens are cow's milk; eggs; fish; shellfish, such as shrimp, crab, and lobster; tree nuts, such as walnuts, almonds, hazelnuts, pecans, cashews, pistachios, and Brazil nuts; peanuts; wheat; soybeans; and sesame.

gut, the immune system in the gut has become quite adept at recognizing what is harmless versus what is dangerous. Some foreign particles can pass through the gut lining and be absorbed into our bloodstream, and our bodies for the most part develop a tolerance. However, in some individuals, the presence of these foreign particles causes the body to rev up its immune system, leading to an allergic reaction.

These immune responses can be divided into those that involve the antibody IgE versus those that do not. Examples of IgE-mediated food allergies include pollen-food allergy syndrome. This is a condition where raw fruits and vegetables lead to itchiness and swelling of the oral cavity. This itchiness and swelling is a result of an IgE response that involves the release of histamine. Other IgE-mediated allergic reactions are not necessarily confined to the oral cavity and can potentially lead to anaphylaxis, a life-threatening, whole-body allergic reaction.

An example of a non-IgE-mediated food allergy is celiac disease, which triggers an immune response to gluten. This leads to the destruction of the intestinal lining, resulting in various symptoms like diarrhea, flatulence, bloating, and sometimes nausea or vomiting. Among infants, there are also conditions like food protein-induced enterocolitis syndrome (FPIES) where various protein sources, especially cow's milk and/or soy protein, can cause an allergic reaction leading to vomiting and diarrhea that disappears once the allergen is removed.

Unlike allergies, food intolerances like lactose or fructose intolerance are not immediately life threatening given the lack of an immune response. Lactose intolerance is a result of reduced production of lactase, the enzyme that helps digest lactose, the sugar that is often found in dairy products like milk and cheese. Again, unlike milk allergies, the symptoms of intolerance do not result in anaphylaxis.

Although not deadly, lactose intolerance can be uncomfortable and lead to dramatic symptoms like profuse diarrhea and weight loss over time. Avoiding dairy products can lead to inadequate calcium and vitamin D intake for those who are not seeking other sources of these nutrients. Nonceliac gluten sensitivity is another food intolerance where gluten seems to trigger certain symptoms even when celiac disease isn't present. The tricky thing is that

The most common allergens among young children include milk, eggs, peanuts, tree nuts, and wheat.

there is no specific test for this condition, and many of these symptoms overlap with other disorders like IBS. In fact, in a third of patients with self-diagnosed gluten sensitivity, an alternative diagnosis was made by a doctor.

The goal of diagnosis is to figure out what foods are causing a reaction, and treatment is essentially avoiding these foods. Typically, IgE-mediated conditions can be diagnosed using a skin prick test or a blood test to detect food-specific IgE. For non-IgE-mediated food allergies, a combination of doing an endoscopy with tissue sampling and blood tests may be required.

As intolerances are not life threatening the way immune-mediated reactions are, trying to avoid certain foods and seeing whether symptoms resolve may be all that is needed to treat the condition. However, if you think you have a food intolerance, the best thing to do is to work with a registered dietitian to identify your triggers and make dietary changes.

ALLERGY LABELING ON PACKAGING

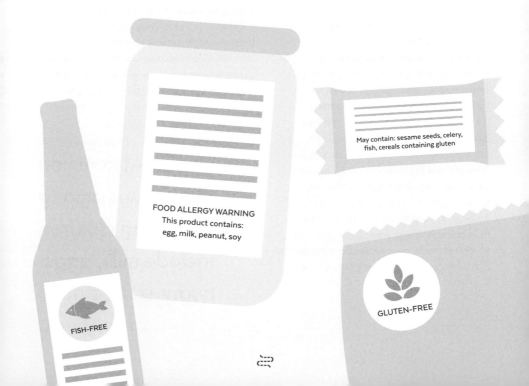

May contain: sesame seeds, celery, fish, cereals containing gluten

FOOD ALLERGY WARNING
This product contains:
egg, milk, peanut, soy

GLUTEN-FREE

FISH-FREE

macronutrients

The body needs macronutrients in large
amounts for energy, growth, and repair.

The three main macronutrients are protein, carbohydrates, and fats. Some foods contain multiple macronutrients, whereas others consist mostly of one macronutrient.

Proteins are large molecules that carry out various functions: providing structure to cells, catalyzing reactions, or transporting molecules between locations in the body. The building blocks of proteins are called amino acids. There are 20 different amino acids, nine of which are considered "essential" as they are not made by the body itself so need to be consumed. Unlike fat and carbohydrates, there is no way for the body to store excess protein. There may be greater protein requirements when the body is under metabolic stress (exercise) or experiencing specific illnesses (burns, protein-losing enteropathy). Common sources of protein include fish, meat, eggs, tofu, and yogurt.

Some carbohydrates are digestible, like starch, sucrose, and lactose, whereas other carbohydrates are indigestible, like soluble and insoluble fiber. When digestible carbohydrates are broken down, they are dismantled into their building blocks of simple sugars (glucose, fructose, galactose). Glucose is metabolized to generate energy for cells, which makes carbohydrates a good source of energy. Common sources of carbohydrates include fruits and vegetables but also starches and cereals. Besides carbohydrates, fruits and vegetables also contain other important nutrients and antioxidants.

Although fats are commonly dismissed as unhealthy substances, many of our bodily functions rely on fats. Lipids, which consist of triglycerides, phospholipids, and cholesterols, serve as sources of energy, components of cell membranes, and precursors to steroid and sex hormones, among other functions. Triglycerides are broken down into glycerol and fatty acids for energy. Like carbohydrates, some dietary sources of fats are considered "healthier" than others. Unlike saturated fats, unsaturated fats (found in high amounts in avocados, nuts, and

Common sources of protein include fish, meat, eggs, tofu, and yogurt.

olive oil) are considered "healthier" because they are liquids at room temperature and, therefore, less likely to clog up our arteries. Unsaturated fats can be further divided into monounsaturated or polyunsaturated fats, both of which are beneficial to heart health. Some healthy fats, like olive oil, contain antioxidants, like polyphenols, that also help with heart health and ageing. One family of polyunsaturated fats are omega-3 fatty acids, which are not generated by the human body and can be obtained only through food. The three main omega-3 fatty acids are eicosapentaenoic acid (EPA) and docosahexaenoic acid (DHA), both found in fish, and alpha-linolenic acid (ALA), most often found in nuts and vegetable oils. Although industrial trans fats (first introduced into foods in the early 20th century to prolong shelf life) are unsaturated fats, they are considered harmful. Commonly found in processed foods, such as cakes, chips, cookies, and margarine, trans fats are considered harmful as they increase the risk of clogged arteries and heart attacks. In 2020, the US banned food manufacturers from adding trans fats to foods. In the UK, there is more a mixed picture, with major brands and retailers agreeing to eliminate trans fats from their products but no specific legislation in place to ban their use.

MACRONUTRIENTS

Proteins, carbohydrates, and fats are the main macronutrients that give our bodies structure and the ability to function. This diagram shows some of the common sources of these macronutrients, and fortunately many foods are a combination of more than one.

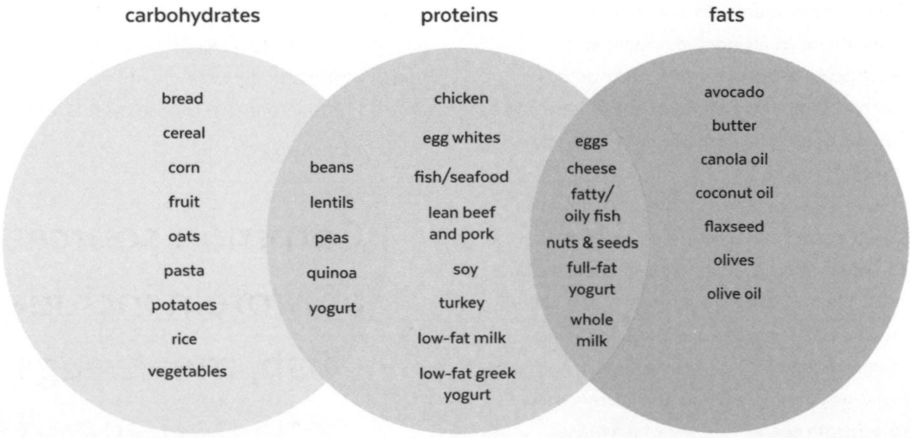

carbohydrates

bread
cereal
corn
fruit
oats
pasta
potatoes
rice
vegetables

beans
lentils
peas
quinoa
yogurt

proteins

chicken
egg whites
fish/seafood
lean beef
and pork
soy
turkey
low-fat milk
low-fat greek
yogurt

eggs
cheese
fatty/
oily fish
nuts & seeds
full-fat
yogurt
whole
milk

fats

avocado
butter
canola oil
coconut oil
flaxseed
olives
olive oil

micronutrients

Needed in smaller amounts, micronutrients are vitamins and minerals, which are essential to health and well-being.

Unlike macronutrients, where the daily requirement is measured in grams, our daily micronutrient need is measured in milligrams or less. Typically, vitamins are organic substances made by plants or animals. Vitamins are either fat-soluble or water-soluble. Vitamins A, D, E, and K are fat-soluble vitamins, which means they require fat to be effectively absorbed by the gut. All other vitamins are water-soluble. In disorders where dietary fat cannot be properly metabolized (like pancreatic insufficiency from chronic pancreatitis), there may be associated deficiencies in these fat-soluble vitamins.

Minerals, on the other hand, are inorganic substances, meaning they are naturally found in the soil. There are two types of minerals: macrominerals and trace minerals. Macrominerals (potassium, sodium, magnesium, phosphorus, calcium) are sometimes not considered micronutrients because they are required in slightly greater quantities. A prolonged deficiency of any one vitamin or mineral can lead to serious health consequences.

To function, our bodies require both water-soluble and fat-soluble vitamins. Certain gut illnesses can directly impair the absorption of certain vitamins, leading to deficiencies and resulting symptoms. A healthy whole food diet should contain most, if not all, of the vitamins listed in the chart below. In developed regions around the world, a deficiency in a healthy individual of a single vitamin is uncommon, and a severe deficiency is rare.

DIETARY SOURCES OF YOUR DAILY VITAMINS

VITAMINS	DIETARY SOURCES	DEFICIENCY
A	Meats, eggs, seafood, carrots, pumpkin, spinach	Poor vision, loss of vision at night
D	Fortified milk and cereals, fatty fish	Weak bones (osteomalacia)
E	Vegetable oils, leafy greens, whole grains, nuts	Anemia and neurological problems (rare)

K	Eggs, milk, kale, spinach, broccoli	Bleeding (rare)
C	Citrus fruits, potatoes, spinach, tomatoes	Poor wound healing; if severe: fatigue, depression, connective tissue problems (scurvy)
B1 (thiamine)	Soy milk, ham, watermelon, squash	Irritability, fatigue, heart failure, neurological problems (Wernicke's encephalopathy) and hallucinations (Korsakoff psychosis)
B2 (riboflavin)	Dairy, enriched grains and cereals	Edema, stomatitis, dermatitis
B3 (niacin)	Meats, fish, fortified grains, mushrooms	Dermatitis, diarrhea, dementia (Pellagra)
B5 (pantothenic acid)	Chicken, whole grains, broccoli, avocado pear	Stomatitis, glossitis, depression, confusion, anemia
B6 (pyridoxine)	Meat, fish, legumes, soybeans, bananas	Altered mental state, myalgias, poor appetite, dermatitis, alopecia (rare to have in isolation)
B7 (biotin)	Eggs, soybeans, fish, whole grains	Megaloblastic anemia, nerve dysfunction
B9 (folate)	Leafy greens, beans, fruits, whole grains	Anemia, fatigue, weakness
B12 (cobalamin)	Meat, fish, dairy, fortified cereals	Fatigue, abdominal pain, vomiting (rare to have in isolation)

Deficiencies

For most people, eating a balanced whole food diet should be adequate in providing the necessary micronutrients to maintain good health. However, certain supplements are recommended for some groups of people. Diseased portions of the gut in conditions like inflammatory bowel disease might not properly absorb micronutrients and can result in deficiencies in iron, B12, vitamin D, vitamin K, and more. Depending on which deficiencies are present, supplementation may be necessary to maintain normal levels of these micronutrients. If you're pregnant or trying for a baby, a daily folic acid supplement is recommended by the American College of Obstetricians and Gynecologists and by The National Institute for Health and Care Excellence (NICE). During the winter months when sun exposure is limited, a daily supplement containing 10 micrograms of vitamin D is recommended for everyone, especially babies and children and the elderly and housebound. For people on a plant-based diet or people aged 50 or older, vitamin B12 supplementation is advised because B12 does not occur naturally in plants and absorption declines with age. The most common micronutrient deficiency in the world is iron, often the result of chronic blood loss (especially in women with heavy periods). In developing countries, parasites are a common cause of iron deficiency.

The gut is responsible for absorbing the minerals that are necessary to help our bodies function normally. Macrominerals like sodium and calcium are involved in nerve and muscle function, as well as contributing to the structure of our bones. Microminerals are important for our immune function and metabolism.

DIETARY SOURCES OF YOUR DAILY MACROMINERALS

MACROMINERALS	DIETARY SOURCES	DEFICIENCY
Sodium	Salt, vegetables	Weakness, dehydration
Potassium	Fruit, some vegetables, nuts, fish, meat	Weakness, arrhythmias, paresthesia
Magnesium	Spinach, legumes, seeds, wholewheat bread	Weakness, twitching, arrhythmias

Phosphorus	Red meat, poultry, seafood, legumes, nuts	Weakness, fatigue, heart failure, immune dysfunction
Calcium	Dairy, leafy greens, fish, fortified cereals and soya bean products	Osteomalacia, arrhythmias

DIETARY SOURCES OF YOUR DAILY MICROMINERALS

MICROMINERALS	DIETARY SOURCES	DEFICIENCY
Chromium	Meat, poultry, fish, cheese, nuts	Blood sugar dysregulation, neuropathy, confusion
Copper	Shellfish, nuts, beans, seeds, wholegrain products	Depigmentation of skin and hair, neurological disturbances, skeletal abnormalities, poor wound healing, low immune cell count
Fluoride	Fish, teas	Dental cavities
Iodine	Iodized salt, seafood, some vegetables and grains	Goiter, hypothyroidism. Fetal abnormalities in pregnant women
Iron	Dark leafy green vegetables, red meat, nuts, beans, fortified bread and cereals	Anemia, fatigue
Selenium	Organ meat, seafood, walnuts	Muscle ache, cardiac problems
Zinc	Meat, shellfish, legumes, wholegrains	Growth arrest, infertility, poor wound healing, diarrhea, hair loss, dermatitis

energy metabolism

This biological process describes how your body
tries to meet its nutritional needs to stay alive.

For our organs to properly function, we need energy. Having a way to store this energy is also important because what we consume isn't always consistent. The most efficient stored energy source, triglycerides, is stored in adipose tissue (fat cells). Glycogen, the stored form of glucose in the liver and muscle tissue, is a less efficient energy source but can fuel certain cells, including bone marrow, red and white blood cells, eye tissues, and peripheral nerves, which cannot process fats and require glucose as their fuel source. Of course, energy is only one part of the equation in keeping our bodies healthy and functioning; micronutrients are another.

Many people think of energy balance in the context of weight gain or loss, but it really describes how much energy is consumed and expended (burned). Total energy expenditure can be split into three main categories: resting energy (also known as basal metabolic rate), physical activity, and the thermic effect of food.

Resting energy expenditure is how much energy our bodies need to be awake while doing nothing. Even though the brain, heart, intestines, liver, and kidneys account for just 10 percent of our total body weight, they spend 75 percent of our resting energy expenditure. Different organs require different amounts of energy at rest, and when people are ill or specific organs are diseased, these energy requirements change. While third-degree burns affecting large portions of the body have the greatest energy requirements among medical conditions, severe infections and acute pancreatitis also increase energy demands significantly. Depending on what medical conditions different individuals have, there may be differences not only in the total calories required but also the different macronutrients and micronutrients needed. For instance, patients with kidney failure requiring dialysis need more protein than those who do not.

Energy expenditure of physical activity is the energy spent on both exercise and our daily activities such as standing or walking. The energy required to process the food that we eat falls into another category called the thermic effect of food. Many people forget that our body requires energy to carry out digestion, too!

The energy that we spend to maintain organ function and to keep up with the energy spent in physical activity or processing food is measured in calories. Similarly, the food we consume contains a certain number of calories. Achieving a balance between calories consumed and calories spent by our bodies is what ultimately leads to a stable and healthy weight.

BURNING ENERGY

This piechart shows the daily amount, by per cent, of energy burned by the three main energy expenditure categories in a healthy person with a sedentary to moderately active lifestyle.

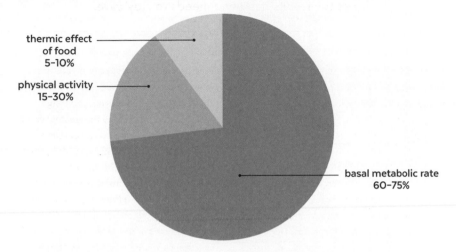

thermic effect
of food
5-10%

physical activity
15-30%

basal metabolic rate
60-75%

ORGAN ENERGY NEEDS

This piechart shows the energy expenditure of individual organs in a healthy person with a sedentary to moderately active lifestyle.

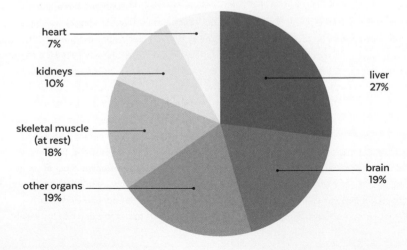

heart
7%

kidneys
10%

skeletal muscle
(at rest)
18%

other organs
19%

liver
27%

brain
19%

Q: CAN I GET SICK FROM TAKING TOO MANY VITAMIN AND MINERAL SUPPLEMENTS?

A: Certain vitamins when taken in excess, typically in concentrated supplemental form, can lead to problems. High doses of vitamin A (retinol) have been shown to increase the risk of lung cancer. Excess vitamin D may cause high levels of calcium in the blood which can lead to nausea, vomiting, bone pain, and kidney problems.

—

Q: IS CONSUMING FAT BAD?

A: As our understanding of fat has changed over time, we have learned that fats are an important element of various parts of the structure and function of the human body. There are both "good" and "bad" fats, and avoiding saturated fats in favor of healthy unsaturated fats can help us reap the benefits of good fats while reducing our risk of cardiovascular disease.

—

Q: SHOULD I NEVER EAT CAKE, COOKIES, OR SWEETS?

A: These foods can be consumed in moderation. Avoiding these foods altogether may lead to cravings that are more difficult to manage in the long run and therefore prove counterproductive.

—

Q: WILL EATING LESS AND OPTING FOR "HEALTHY" FOODS HELP ME LOSE WEIGHT?

A: Choosing foods that are nutrient-rich and less calorie dense that provide a sensation of fullness can help people lose weight without feeling hungry. Some "healthy" foods can still be quite calorie dense. Nuts, for instance, have lots of healthy fats and many other nutritious benefits, but they can be calorie dense and may work against achieving the proper energy balance for weight loss.

—

Q: IS PLANT PROTEIN AS GOOD AS ANIMAL PROTEIN?

A: It's a common misconception that plant proteins are incomplete proteins. In fact, some plant proteins, like quinoa, are complete proteins meaning they contain all nine essential amino acids that must be consumed through our diet. Consuming a diet rich in plant foods may also have the added benefit of having fewer calories, more fiber, and more antioxidants and other micronutrients not found in meat.

———

Q: WILL EATING AND DRINKING SOY PRODUCTS INCREASE MY RISK OF BREAST CANCER?

A: Some animal studies have shown that high doses of plant estrogens found in soy may stimulate breast tumor cell growth. However, this hasn't been observed in human studies. In fact, soy-based foods may have a protective effect.

———

Q: IS EATING A GLUTEN-FREE DIET HEALTHIER?

A: Without a medical reason like celiac disease, avoiding gluten might not confer any health benefit. In fact, limiting foods that contain gluten may lead to missing out on certain key nutrients that are often found in whole grains.

———

Q: IS TAKING A WEIGHT LOSS MEDICATION OR UNDERGOING A WEIGHT LOSS PROCEDURE CHEATING?

A: Weight loss medications and procedures help people lose weight. However, they are not a cure-all solution, nor are they considered "cheating" when it comes to pursuing the health benefits of weight loss. Obesity is often a chronic condition influenced by many external factors beyond an individual's control and should be addressed in a multifaceted approach.

———

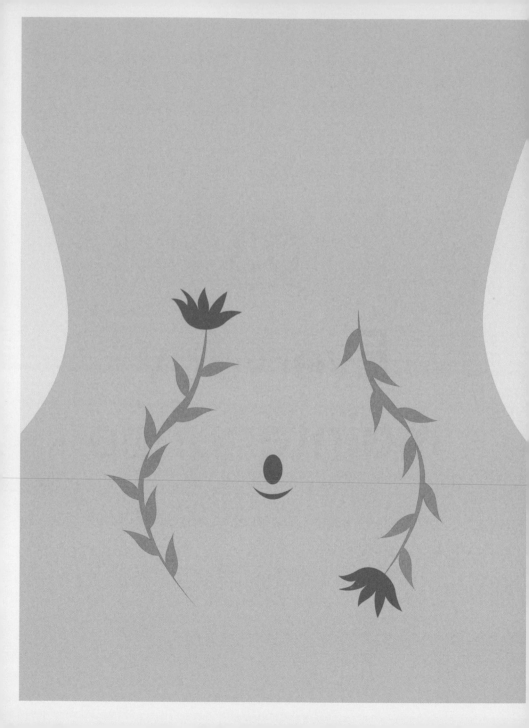

03

Everyday maintenance

what should I eat?

Your doctor has recommended that you
follow a "healthy diet." Now what?

Everyone seems to have a different definition of a "healthy diet." Depending on age, culture, location, and what food is available locally, the definition could range from simply finding food that is uncontaminated and safe to selecting food that fulfills a specific nutritional goal. Eating a diverse diet and choosing whole foods is a great place to start. In recent decades, ultra processed foods have become a significant part of many people's diets. We often trade convenience for limited nutritional value.

According to the World Health Organization (WHO), a healthy diet for adults typically includes fresh fruits and vegetables, legumes, nuts, and whole grains. The WHO recommends consuming at least 400g of fruits and vegetables per day plus 25g of dietary fiber from natural sources. It goes on to recommend that we reduce our total fat consumption to less than 30 percent of our total energy intake (66 grams for a 2,000-calorie-a-day diet) and ensure that our intake of added sugar contributes less than 10 percent of our total energy intake (22 grams for a 2,000-calorie daily intake), with l ess than 5g of salt consumed per day. However, these recommendations can be difficult to measure and visualize. In 2011, the US Department of Agriculture (USDA) launched MyPlate, a more practical visual tool to help people understand how to balance the food groups on a plate. Even MyPlate is not perfect as it doesn't explicitly talk about healthy fats, for instance. Making overnight changes to fit these recommendations is also impractical and at times too drastic.

In recent decades, ultra processed foods have become a significant part of many people's diets.

A great way to start is by making changes gradually, one step at a time. Understanding how much of each food group should go on your plate is the first step, followed by choosing items from each group then preparing them in a healthy way. Doing your own food shopping and preparing meals yourself gives you the most control over what goes into your food. Once at the supermarket, it takes a bit more time (and math) to read nutrition labels to understand what is in your food and to figure out how many calories it contains.

Daily guide

The food pyramid is a thing of the past, and MyPlate is a general guide for how to divide different food groups in a meal on your plate. Having an appropriate balance of these food groups can help ensure you are receiving all the nutrients your body needs to fulfill nutritional requirements while reducing less healthy options. This plate format helps account for differences in caloric needs by age.

FIVE FOOD GROUPS

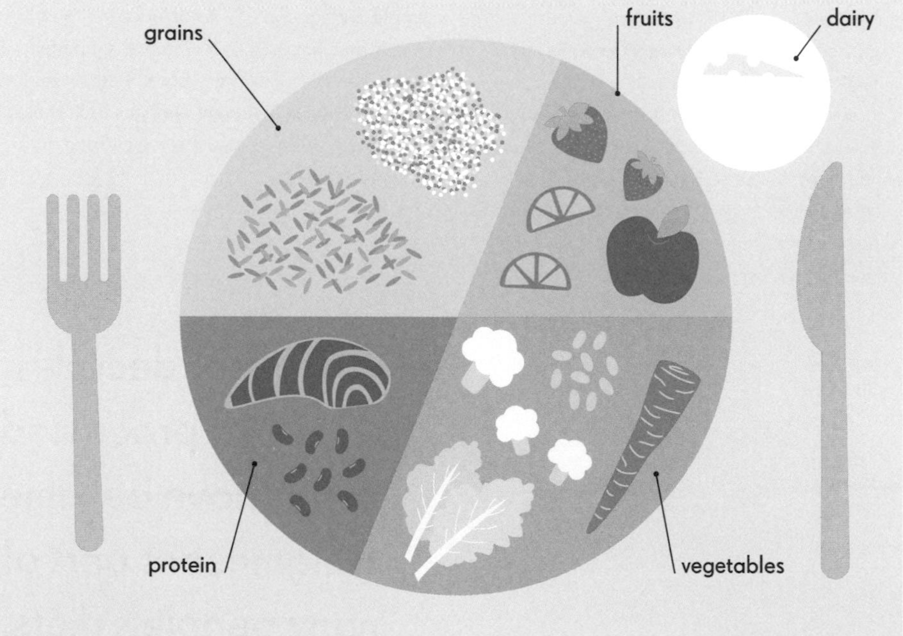

grains

fruits

dairy

protein

vegetables

Food labeling

How food is labeled differs from country to country. Historically in the United States, the Food and Drug Administration (FDA) has required 15 nutrition components to be declared on the panel. These include calories—calories from fat, total fat, saturated fat, and trans fat—plus cholesterol, sodium, carbohydrates, dietary fiber, sugars, protein, vitamin A, vitamin C, calcium, and iron. However, with our current understanding that the *type* of fat is more important than the *amount* of fat consumed, the FDA recently removed "calories from fat" from the list of components required on food labels, along with vitamin A and vitamin C (given how rare deficiencies in these vitamins are today). They also recently updated labeling to display serving size and total calories per serving in a larger font, and labels should now show "added sugars" as well as vitamin D and potassium.

Reading the small print

Understanding how to read a nutrition label is important in order to know what macronutrients and micronutrients we are consuming and how much is in each serving. This is particularly helpful if you are looking to reduce your intake of saturated fat or limit the amount of salt consumed.

TRAFFIC-LIGHT LABELLING

In the UK, supermarkets and some food manufacturers add a traffic-light label to prepackaged food packaging. Green means that a certain nutrient is low, amber means medium, and red is high in a nutrient. In this way we know what foods we should avoid, eat less often, or eat in smaller amounts.

Each ½ pack serving contains

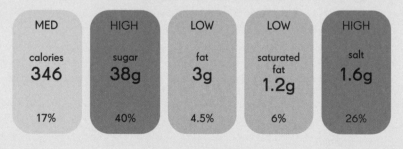

MED	HIGH	LOW	LOW	HIGH
calories	sugar	fat	saturated fat	salt
346	38g	3g	1.2g	1.6g
17%	40%	4.5%	6%	26%

Beyond calories and nutrients, other labels are put on food packaging too; some of these labels are helpful, others less so. One example is how eggs are graded. In the US, eggs are graded AA, A, and B based on how thick the egg whites are and how strong the shells are. Other labels indicate the conditions in which the hens live. Eggs labeled "free-range" are laid by hens that have access to the outdoors, and hens that are "pasture-raised" can graze naturally on pasture (although there is no official definition of what makes a pasture). Eggs labeled "cage-free" do not necessarily mean cruelty-free, and "all natural" or "farm fresh" have no clear meaning. Even labels like "no hormones" or "vegetarian fed" may be misleading, as hens are natural omnivores and in the US are not given hormones.

Claims like "naturally sweetened" are not well defined, and other labels like "fair trade" or "vegan" may be certified by third-party organizations and difficult to verify. There are also subtle differences in claims, including the USDA Organic seal versus those that simply state "organic" on the packaging. All these nuances in labeling makes it difficult to discern what products and foods to select. Also, many of these labels are not enforced by a regulatory body. In the US, there are multiple federal agencies responsible for regulating various foods, including the USDA, FDA, and local water departments and public health agencies. It can be quite confusing since the USDA regulates meat, poultry, and egg products, the FDA regulates many other food items, while the public health agencies regulate restaurant businesses.

• USE-BY AND BEST-BEFORE DATES •

Use by is the key date in terms of safety and can be seen on food that goes off quickly, such as meat, fish, milk, and prepackaged salads and vegetables. Do not eat food after the use-by date.

Best before is more about quality than safety and is typically found on foods that are dried, canned, or frozen. Food is still safe to eat after the best-before date but may lose quality, in terms of flavor and texture. Eggs, however, should be eaten before the best-before date.

kitchen hygiene

How food is prepared, cooked, and stored
can impact your gut health.

Food prep

There are various ways of cooking foods such as grilling, baking, frying, air frying, smoking, roasting, and steaming. Some methods are healthier than others. Research has shown that by-products of deep-fried foods can trigger inflammation, exacerbating existing inflammatory conditions and increasing the risk of other diseases. Advanced glycation end-products (AGEs) are commonly linked to oxidative stress at the cellular level, contributing to a range of health conditions such as diabetes and cancer. AGEs not only are associated with insulin resistance but can also reduce gut microbiota diversity and beneficial metabolites. Furthermore, deep-frying food can inadvertently add extra calories as more fat is absorbed, especially in foods covered in batter, which is unhelpful for those with obesity or diabetes. Other methods of cooking such as smoking or charring can damage foods and introduce to the body harmful cancer-causing compounds known as carcinogens. Some studies have shown that well-done, grilled meat has been

linked to a 19 percent increase in the risk of precancerous adenomatous polyps, the precursors of colorectal cancer. There are many foods, especially fruits and vegetables, that can be enjoyed uncooked or lightly steamed, preserving more nutrients and avoiding the use of cooking oils.

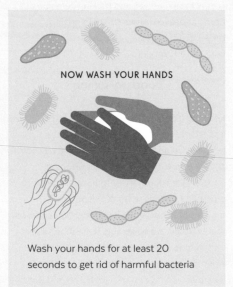

NOW WASH YOUR HANDS

Wash your hands for at least 20 seconds to get rid of harmful bacteria

Contamination

Proper handwashing prior to food preparation and separating raw meat from other raw produce will help avoid contamination. Good hygiene practices before cooking can prevent foodborne illnesses caused by pathogens like *Listeria, Salmonella*, and *E. Coli*. For greens, such as salad bags, that have been prewashed, it is recommended not to wash again to reduce the risk of further contamination from contact with the sink, your hands, or other surrounding items. For grocery deliveries or delivered meal kits, getting to know your vendor, understanding their hygiene practices, ensuring the packaging is intact upon arrival, and making sure you are home at delivery times can help prevent the food from spoiling when not refrigerated properly.

Food poisoning

Ensuring leftovers are handled properly is important to staying healthy. Adequate refrigeration and reheating can be the difference between safe dining and food poisoning. Food that is left out in room temperature for prolonged periods or is not adequately reheated may result in bacterial growth and harbor toxins that lead to food poisoning. Reheating soups and sauces to a boil is a good practice. Also, when dining out, don't ask for a doggy bag if your plan is not to go straight home and put the leftovers in a fridge.

Cleaning

When cleaning up after a meal, it's important to use proper cleaning materials and tools. For example, wire grill brushes are not recommended for cleaning grills because bristles can potentially be left on the grill and inadvertently swallowed, lodging in the esophagus, resulting in a medical emergency. Using damaged cooking or cleaning utensils or having an old cutting board that can harbor bacteria and trapped particles may also cause health problems.

• HIGH-RISK FOODS •

Any type of food can cause food poisoning, but there are certain foods that are more likely to make you sick.

• Raw and undercooked meat, poultry, and eggs

• Unwashed raw fruits and vegetables

• Raw seafood

• Raw milk and products made from it, including raw soft cheeses

• Leafy greens, including prepackaged salads

• Raw or undercooked sprouts, such as alfalfa sprouts or bean sprouts

fiber-a-day

Fiber is a type of complex carbohydrate
that our bodies cannot digest.

Found naturally in plant foods, fiber includes compounds such as cellulose, hemicellulose, and pectin, among others. Eating an adequate amount of dietary fiber every day can help promote regularity of bowel movements, improve stool consistency, and even reduce cholesterol absorption. Fiber does not get completely digested by digestive enzymes, and the undigested fiber undergoes fermentation in the large intestine, where it encounters gut microbiota. The degree to which fermentation occurs can impact the amount of gas that is produced and the potential discomfort experienced by some. Unfortunately, many people who seek solutions from fiber consumption also suffer from gut issues, such as IBS, which can be made worse by fiber. Fiber comes in various forms. Soluble fiber dissolves in water, whereas insoluble fiber does not. Many foods contain a combination of the two types of fiber, and soluble fiber tends to help with stool consistency whereas insoluble fiber helps with bulking up the stool.

TWO TYPES OF FIBER

Soluble fiber		Insoluble fiber	
artichoke	banana	brown rice	seeds
garlic	onion	some legumes	vegetables
soybeans	wheat	celery	quinoa

Everyone has a unique gut microbiota and, therefore, reacts to foods in different ways. If bloating is an issue for you, it is important to first rule out other causes like constipation or food sensitivities, which can be treated in other ways. Instead of eliminating high-fiber foods entirely, try to identify which foods are most likely to trigger bloating, gassiness, and abdominal pain. This process of elimination is important as you can then avoid specific high-fiber foods that trigger symptoms while enjoying the nutritious benefits of others. Many complex carbohydrates, including fruits and vegetables, contain both fiber and prebiotics—compounds that play an important role in the health of gut microbiota. If these foods are avoided out of fear of developing symptoms, a vicious cycle might result as the microbiota would be deprived of these prebiotic foods.

What is the difference between pre- and probiotics?

Prebiotics are foods, mainly nondigestible fibers, that help stimulate the growth and activity of beneficial bacteria in the large intestine. These bacteria ferment prebiotics, creating short-chain fatty acids, which are beneficial to our health. However, not all dietary fiber contains prebiotics. Some natural sources of prebiotics include raw chicory root, raw dandelion greens, raw leek, raw asparagus, and human breast milk. Many prebiotic supplements contain a mix of fiber or fruit or vegetable derivatives.

Probiotics, on the other hand, describe live bacteria that when given in sufficient amounts offer a health benefit. Anecdotal evidence has shown traditional fermented foods and drinks, like kimchi, sauerkraut, kombucha, or miso, that contain "live and active" bacteria confer some health benefits, but scientific evidence to prove this probiotic benefit is limited. Some fermented foods undergo a degree of processing, like baking or canning, that may render inactive the probiotics. There are many over-the-counter probiotic supplements available but not all have documented health benefits. While many people may benefit from such supplements, some will not. Typically, scientific studies look at specific species and strains of bacteria administered in different amounts in a clinical setting, making it difficult to offer specific probiotic recommendations to individuals.

• FIBER AND IBD •

A low-fiber diet is often recommended for IBD patients to reduce the risk of obstructing an intestinal stricture. However, there is little evidence to demonstrate any benefit in this, whether during a flare or not. In fact, some scientists argue that the anti-inflammatory properties of short-chain fatty acids would benefit patients with IBD.

food modifications

Modifications to our food and added synthetic extras
are subject to a lot of controversy. Let's explore the main
contenders and their pros and cons.

Genetically modified organisms (GMOs)

For centuries, humans have crossbred plants. Gregor Mendel, who first described the basics of genetics, was able to do so after breeding two different types of peas in 1866. Genetic engineering, or biotechnology, uses scientific techniques to speed up the process of genetic modification, allowing breeders to select beneficial traits (drought and herbicide tolerance, disease and insect resistance) to help prevent crop loss and produce greater yields. This enables farmers to use fewer pesticides and till the soil less (to prevent weeds) and maintain soil health. GMO crops include corn, soybeans, potato, sugar beet, and rice. Some scientists argue that GMOs come with risks to the environment such as reducing biodiversity in areas surrounding crops, impacting native insect and plant species.

GM food describes food developed from genetically modified organisms. In the US, more than 90 percent of corn, cotton, and soy come from GMO seeds, meaning that much of the food eaten is likely to contain GMOs. Altering plant genes can slow the rate of spoiling, which can prolong the shelf life of GM foods, thereby reducing food waste. As GMO crops are easier and less costly to grow, GM foods often are cheaper to buy. While some studies have reported no harmful effects on human health from eating GM foods, others have raised concerns about health risks such as altering the gut microbiome and triggering immune reactions, notably allergies.

Antibiotics

One of the most important innovations in the history of medicine, antibiotics allow us to fight off previously life-threatening infections. But overuse of antibiotics across populations and in animal husbandry has caused issues. In addition to treating infections in livestock, some antibiotics have been used to promote faster growth in certain animals, like chickens. Since 2017, antibiotic use has significantly changed after the US banned antibiotics for production purposes and started requiring veterinarian prescriptions for disease-specific antibiotics.

While some people remain concerned about antibiotic resistance and other potential health problems like rare allergic reactions and alterations of the gut microbiota (link still unclear), others continue to doubt whether exposure to low levels of antibiotic residue is responsible. However, nowadays with strict regulations and required testing, antibiotics are largely prevented from entering the food supply.

Monosodium glutamate (MSG)

Used to enhance the flavor of processed, canned, and frozen foods, MSG is a common food additive. Some manufacturers use it to reduce salt in foods, which may be helpful for those with cardiovascular disease. MSG is created by fermenting plants to create glutamate and then adding sodium to create crystals that look like salt. According to the FDA, MSG is "generally recognized as safe." Some people report being sensitive to MSG, reporting headaches and digestive discomfort. But there's still not much evidence to confirm a link.

Food coloring and dyes

Synthetic food dyes are petroleum-based substances used to give some food items a certain color. Currently, the FDA approves nine food dyes, including Red 40, Yellow 5, and Yellow 6, which can be found in many foods and drinks such as breakfast cereals, candy, chips, and soft drinks. There are some concerns about the impact of synthetic food dyes on health, notably a possible association with cancer, although scientific evidence is limited (with no evidence in humans, specifically). Nonetheless, several US states are looking into proactively banning certain dyes. Since foods using these dyes are often of little nutritional value, the general recommendation is to avoid these foods even if the dye itself is not defined as harmful. Some manufacturers have replaced synthetic dyes with dyes derived from plants, animals, and minerals.

•WHAT IS PROCESSED FOOD? •

Processed food is any product from the farm that has been changed from its natural state. Think frozen vegetables. However, not all processed foods are the same. Some foods are "ultra" processed, meaning they have been through multiple processes and transformed by using five or more ingredients, additives, and ingredients not typically found in your kitchen at home.

Sweeteners

Sugar substitutes and sweeteners include aspartame, sucralose, saccharin, as well as plant-based sweeteners like stevia. Many of these sugar alternatives have been developed to provide more sweetness from smaller amounts. Sweeteners are often used as sugar substitutes because they do not raise blood sugar or directly contribute calories in the way sugar does. For those looking to lose weight, using sweeteners may help. However, sweeteners are often found in ultra-processed foods that have little to no nutritional benefit. Some researchers even suggest that their use may enhance sugar cravings and be counterproductive for those with conditions such as obesity.

Developed in the mid-20th century, high-fructose corn syrup (HFCS) is a sweetener made from corn starch. Cheaper and easier to manufacture compared to granulated sugar, HFCS is often found in sweetened foods and drinks. Concerns have been raised about its contribution toward fatty deposits in the liver, leading some food manufacturers and restaurants to remove HFCS from their products.

Preservatives

Preservatives describe substances used to prevent food decomposition. Some preservatives (like nitrates and benzoates) have antimicrobial properties to prevent bacterial degradation, while others are antioxidants to prevent fats from going rancid. Concerns around preservatives are often country-specific, and the benefits and risks of using them are viewed differently. For instance, some developing countries rely on these preservatives to mitigate food scarcity.

Nitrates

Composed of nitrogen and oxygen atoms, nitrates (NO_3) are compounds found naturally in the human body and in dark leafy green vegetables. Nitrates are added to meats, fish, and other foods to help prevent the growth of bacteria, add flavor, and preserve the pink/red color of meats. Foods highest in nitrates include cured meats like ham, bacon, and deli meat. Bacteria and enzymes in the gut convert nitrates to nitrites (NO_2), which react with amines in meat to create nitrosamines, a potential carcinogen. Increasingly, the use of nitrates in processed meats has come under scrutiny. Some studies have shown that more of these nitrosamines are generated by cooking these meats in high heat. These findings have led some governments to remove, where possible, the use of nitrates in food production. Also, eating processed meats comes with the additional concerns of high sodium levels and other additives. Although leafy greens also contain nitrates, these vegetables have other compounds and antioxidants that prevent nitrosamine formation and can have an overall positive effect on the body, notably on cardiovascular health.

Plant-based meat

Derived from soybeans, peas, or wheat, and often marketed as an alternative to meat, plant-based meats have gained in popularity. While these products bring environmental and animal welfare benefits, the health advantages of these substitutes have been called into question. Although reducing red meat consumption is generally encouraged, these plant-based meats are often highly processed and contain added sugars, coloring, and bulking agents. If you are concerned about reducing your intake of highly processed foods but want to maintain a plant-based diet, tofu, tempeh, beans, pulses, and mushrooms can offer healthier alternatives and still provide the desired texture and flavor of meat.

Sweeteners are often found in ultra-processed foods that have little to no nutritional benefit.

let's get physical

There is growing evidence to suggest that exercise
may have positive effects on the gut microbiota.

Independent of diet, some studies describe a shift in the gut microbiota population with physical activity to favor better bacterial groups. Other studies have specifically demonstrated an increase in short-chain fatty acids. These short-chain fatty acids may have anti-inflammatory properties that could benefit various gastrointestinal conditions.

Exercise may also have different effects on our gut microbiota at different stages in life. Some animal studies suggest that exercise early in life has greater influences on microbiota composition. Perhaps this could be a result of physical activity outdoors as some evidence suggests that contact with soil may alter gut microbial diversity early in life. Given emerging evidence of the gut-brain connection, exercise-induced differences in the gut microbiota may also have an impact on mental health. Some scientists even suggest a possibility for gut microbes to influence our motivation to exercise by producing metabolites that stimulate dopamine levels that activate reward and motivation centers in the brain.

Other organs in the gastrointestinal (GI) system can also benefit from physical activity. The effect of exercise on the pancreas may benefit patients with diabetes. Some of these effects include changes in blood flow to the pancreas, stimulation of pancreatic cells, and hormone secretion (including insulin, glucagon, and somatostatin). Both aerobic and resistance exercise (anaerobic) have been shown to improve liver fat content, and physical activity in general appears to slow the progression of fatty liver disease. While the exact quantity of physical activity is not known, according to the American College of Sports Medicine (ACSM), at least 150 min/week of moderate or 75 min/week of vigorous-intensity physical activity is recommended for patients with metabolic associated steatotic liver disease (nonalcoholic fatty liver disease).

• CAUGHT SHORT •

The relationship between physical activity and gut health can be clearly demonstrated in athletes. For example, runner's diarrhea is a condition caused by excess stimulation of the intestines, notably gut motility, and reduced circulation to certain parts of the gut, which causes intestinal inflammation and bleeding. This condition resolves on its own, if the exercise intensity is reduced.

BENEFITS OF GETTING PHYSICAL

Helps keep
you regular

Promotes healthy
gut bacteria

Improves
blood circulation

Reduces chronic inflammation

Lowers risk of colon cancer

Lowers stress level

Decreases weight

Reduces liver fat content

On the other end of the spectrum, another example of how physical activity is linked to gut transit time is in those who are hospitalized or bedbound. Rates of constipation are much higher in these patients, especially if these patients are taking narcotic pain medications after surgery, which can further slow the gut. At times in the hospital, nursing staff are sometimes instructed to rotate the patient at regular intervals to help promote bowel movements.

In the happy medium of low to moderate-intensity exercise, the reduced gut transit time may move toxins along more quickly in the gut, limiting exposure to the gut lining. Beyond identifying the relationship between physical activity and gut transit, exercise has also been shown to have significant benefits for a variety of conditions, including various cancers (including colon cancer) and cardiovascular disease.

stress and the gut

Stress can trigger a wide range of gastrointestinal
problems and exacerbate existing gut diseases, too.

The gut-brain axis describes the bidirectional communication between the gut and the brain, and specifically how the gut microbiota affects this interaction. Emotional stress is a a normal response comparable to worry, frustration, sadness, and fear that everyone experiences on occasion in response to difficult situations. However, when this mental state becomes so severe or chronic that it begins to interfere with daily activities, there may be a specific psychiatric diagnosis at play such as generalized anxiety disorder or obsessive compulsive disorder (OCD).

Understanding how emotional stress relates to the gut microbiota has been of particular interest to many scientists. Although chronic emotional stress has been linked to inflammatory bowel disease flares, only recently has there been evidence describing the mechanism of how stress not only exacerbates gut symptoms in IBD but also leads to gut inflammation. In 2023, a study found that glial cells (which support neurons) in animals with IBD were shown to deliver stress signals from the brain that led to inflammation in the gut.

• FIGHT OR FLIGHT? •

One way our bodies responds to stress is through a release of neurotransmitters like adrenaline and serotonin. This is most pronounced in an acute fight-or-flight situation. These neurotransmitters get our heart pumping faster and affect our gut function in various ways, including its movement. In fact, some people experience "nervous poops" where they feel the urge to go to the bathroom when they feel nervous or stressed, while others describe soiling their pants when faced with a fight-or-flight situation. Existing literature also suggests that long-term stress may alter the gut-brain interaction in a way that heightens the response in conditions like IBS.

In this study, chronic elevated levels of glucocorticoids such as cortisol led to white blood cells being attracted to the gut, thereby increasing inflammation. Furthermore, the gut nerve cells (of the enteric nervous system) also stopped functioning normally, leading to worsening of IBD symptoms.

The origin of psychiatric conditions like major depressive disorder or anxiety is not well understood, and changes in the gut microbiota have been investigated as a potential culprit. Some researchers have found evidence of different populations of gut bacteria that produce more, or less, butyrate, glutamate, or other by-products that influence the metabolism of neurotransmitters that may affect depression, anxiety, or other psychiatric conditions. However, gut flora cannot reliably predict the presence of these disorders. Moreover, the impact of age and geographic location on gut microbiota in relation to psychiatric conditions is poorly understood. Some researchers have also tried looking into how psychotropic medications (used to treat

BRAIN CHANGE

Stress, genetics, and our upbringing can influence the gut-brain axis, which in turn can affect gut function. When your body is under chronic, long-standing stress, the hardwiring of your brain is altered, which can affect how symptoms are experienced in conditions such as IBS.

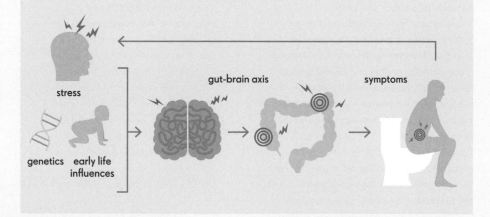

stress

genetics   early life
            influences

gut-brain axis

symptoms

psychiatric conditions) may impact or be influenced by the gut flora. Although this relationship is vague at present, it may be important to understand how differences in individual gut microbes might influence the processing of the drug and impact the efficacy of these medications or how these medications might alter how the gut microbiota function.

Other studies have looked at the potential impact stress has on gut microbiota. Some of these studies have focused on different sources of stress (like in utero, early life, chronic stress) in both animal and human models and found changes in the composition of gut flora. Some of these studies have gone further to draw associations with observed changes in inflammatory responses (like changes in cytokines levels). However, these findings are not conclusive, especially in humans. If more concrete evidence can be generated, the next step would be figuring out how to adjust diet and influence the gut microbiota in a way that may modify the effect of stress.

Some studies in both animal and humans have even suggested an effect of stress on the gut microbiota across generations. Maternal stress during certain periods of pregnancy has been linked to reduced microbial diversity in the newborn. Whether these changes result in downstream inflammatory responses or other long-term reactions remains unknown.

The relationship between stress and inflammation in the gut is complex because the gut-brain axis is bidirectional. Inflammation in the gut also signals back to the brain, further contributing to anxiety and depression-like responses. In fact, studies have shown that

patients with active inflammatory bowel disease seem to experience more anxiety and depression than those with inactive disease. Recognizing this relationship between the gut and the brain can potentially help patients cope by providing an organic explanation.

While there are likely many contributors to mental health, the gut may play a key role in this complex process. The hope is that one day we will have targeted strategies and medications that can help alter the gut microbiome to prevent and treat a wide variety of ailments, including mental health conditions.

Stress during certain periods of pregnancy has been linked to reduced microbial diversity in the newborn.

babies, children, and teens

Pediatric gastroenterology is a subspeciality
focused on gastrointestinal conditions in
babies, children, and teenagers.

Some babies and children have anatomic malformations where the gut fails to develop in the womb as expected. A few of these malformations are isolated to the gut, while other abnormalities are part of broader developmental syndromes such as Down syndrome. Abnormal development of gut organs can be debilitating and may require surgical repair. While some abnormalities are structural (disorder in anatomy), others are functional. For example, esophageal atresia is a structural defect as the esophagus is connected to the airway (trachea), which can cause swallowed liquid to travel into the lungs, leading to lung infections (pneumonia). Hirschsprung's disease is a functional condition where nerve cells are missing from the large intestine, causing severe constipation and bowel distention because the intestine isn't passing stools. Often surgery is required within days of birth to remove the affected part of the colon.

In the first years of life, young children are less able to verbalize their concerns, and gut problems may appear in unusual ways. Without the ability to accurately describe how they're feeling, children with constipation may demonstrate irritability or fecal soiling. Babies with gastroesophageal reflux disorder (GERD) may not display symptoms common to GERD, such as regurgitation, but rather show poor growth and irritability. Diagnosing GERD in babies can be particularly challenging as a symptom like regurgitation is often normal at this age.

Young children are less able to verbalize their concerns, and gut problems may appear in unusual ways.

Scientists have also identified how breastfeeding may contribute to the development of the gut microbiota early in life. Studies investigating the composition of gut microbes in infants fed with breast milk versus formula found a greater diversity of gut bacteria in breastfed babies. As microbes exist on the skin and are transferred through skin contact, there may be nuances between babies fed from the breast and those fed with milk extracted via a breast pump.

Teenagers

The teenage years can be challenging enough without having a gastrointestinal condition on top. However, it is during adolescence when some GI conditions may first appear, and this can be distressing, especially as seeking a diagnosis and undergoing treatment may have a significant impact on quality of life during a key life stage. Some conditions diagnosed in childhood and teenage years may include celiac disease, eosinophilic esophagitis, inflammatory bowel disease, and food allergies and intolerances. Symptoms associated with these conditions may be exacerbated by the stress and anxiety of coping with the disease at this sensitive time. As a way of coping, acknowledging this difficulty might be the first step in fostering a healthy dialogue between parents and children.

During adolescence, alterations to the gut can happen. The influence of friends, social media, and the potential introduction of unhealthy habits like poor sleep patterns, vaping, or substance misuse may pose a challenge on top of the physiological changes that take place during this transition to adulthood.

How puberty and sex hormones affect the gut microbiota (and vice versa) remains unclear, and even less is known specifically about how the gut and the onset of menstruation are related. Anecdotally, some teens may experience symptoms like nausea, vomiting, or changes in bowel movements with menstrual cycles so the gut and reproductive system may be linked in other ways.

The conversation around weight and healthy eating can also be challenging for teens. As they gain autonomy over their own food choices, they must navigate through this life stage amid peer and societal pressure. Involving children and teens in shopping and decision-making on meal planning can help instill healthy habits early on.

the uterus and the gut

Beyond their proximity to one another, the gut and
the uterus share a special relationship influenced
by hormones and the nervous system.

Endometriosis

Endometriosis describes a condition where cells
that normally line the uterus grow outside of the
uterus. During menstruation, the uterine lining
sloughs off and exits the vagina. Some of these
lining cells can travel in the opposite way, into
the abdominal cavity, and stick onto the outer
surface of the intestines and other organs.
These cells remain active and can bleed with
each menstrual cycle. Endometriosis can
be associated with other symptoms like
constipation, menstrual cramps, painful bowel
movements, nausea, vomiting, diarrhea, rectal
bleeding, or recurrent miscarriage. Pain can
result from irritation of the nerves from the
growing endometriosis itself, irritation from
bleeding into the gut, and inflammation.

Endometriosis can be difficult to diagnose at
times. While it can sometimes be detected on

MIGRATING TISSUES
Endometriosis is a condition where abnormal tissue deposits from the endometrium develop
outside the uterus and can form anywhere around the uterus, including on the bowel. When
this occurs, this can cause abdominal pain and bleeding into the gut, among other symptoms.

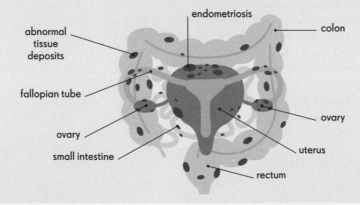

abnormal tissue deposits

endometriosis

colon

fallopian tube

ovary

ovary

small intestine

uterus

rectum

scans, in other instances it may require surgical exploration of the abdomen to diagnose. Treatment may include oral contraceptive pills (or hormones) to regulate the cells.

Menstruation

Experiencing GI symptoms like abdominal pain, nausea, bloating, and diarrhea around your menstrual cycle is common. If you have IBS, you may be more prone to have these symptoms, and sometimes in a more frequent and pronounced way than those who do not have this GI condition. Some hormones that help regulate menstrual cycles may affect certain gut symptoms. For instance, prostaglandins, which are typically released by cells and associated with processes like inflammation, are also in abundance during menstruation (from the destruction of endometrial cells that line the uterus). These prostaglandins are thought to cause fecal incontinence or "period poops" by stimulating the intestinal muscles. Right after ovulation, the hormone progesterone increases dramatically and may cause the opposite effect, slowing the gut down and causing constipation.

Experiencing GI symptoms around your menstrual cycle is common.

Pregnancy

In pregnancy, other GI symptoms are seen at higher rates, including nausea, vomiting, GERD, and constipation. This can be due to a variety of reasons, including fluctuating hormones and an enlarged uterus housing a growing fetus. Nausea and vomiting are the most common conditions, affecting up to 80 percent of women, starting at weeks 4 to 6 and peaking at weeks 8 to 12. While many do not require medication, first-line medical treatments may include histamine receptor blockers like promethazine, since no adverse effects on the fetus have been reported. GERD affects between 40 and 85 percent of pregnant women as well. Apart from simple measures like avoiding late-night meals and elevating the head of the bed, first-line therapy typically consists of antacids, followed by H2 blockers. The safety of proton pump inhibitors has been questioned in the past for use in pregnancy. However, many studies have generally demonstrated safety regarding fetal toxicity.

Hyperemesis gravidarum is a severe form of nausea and vomiting, accompanied by weight loss, dehydration, and electrolyte imbalances thought to be related to hormonal changes during pregnancy. Treatment usually consists of intravenous hydration, vitamins, and anti-nausea medications.

Several diseases affect the liver during pregnancy. Intrahepatic cholestasis of pregnancy occurs because of slowed bile flow from hormonal changes. In late pregnancy, bile acid levels rise, and skin can become jaundiced and itchy. It is generally a benign condition for the mother, although there are risks to the unborn child that typically require delivery by week 37 of gestation.

Liver changes can also appear with preeclampsia (hypertension and proteinuria during pregnancy) or eclampsia (when seizures also occur), which occur in 2 to 8 percent of pregnancies. Changes in circulation may lead to liver dysfunction and cell death, although no specific treatment for the liver is usually required. About 5 to 10 percent of women with severe preeclampsia may also experience complications of life-threatening hemolysis, elevated liver enzymes, and low platelet count, also called HELLP syndrome. In addition to nausea, vomiting, and right upper quadrant pain, severe bleeding and clotting complications may occur. Acute liver failure from HELLP is rare but may require liver transplantation. Acute fatty liver of pregnancy (AFLP) is a disorder in the third trimester where long-chain fatty acids accumulate in the fetal and maternal circulation, which can be deadly and requires urgent delivery and intensive care.

After childbirth, pelvic floor dysfunction is common, and the weakened pelvic floor muscles could increase risk of fecal incontinence and rectal prolapse. While Kegel exercises, meant to strengthen the pelvic floor muscles, may be helpful in some situations, a specialist in pelvic floor physical therapy may need to assess if this is appropriate for you.

Menopause

Menopause is when menstrual cycles end, and sex hormones also typically decline. Our understanding of the effect of these hormonal changes on gut symptoms is still limited. Some researchers have shown that in patients with IBS, symptoms can become magnified after menopause, possibly due to the low levels of progesterone and estradiol. Researchers believe that the absence of these hormones can affect the nervous system and how pain is perceived. How the reduction in these sex hormones affects the gut microbiota is another area of study. There is some evidence to suggest lower overall diversity of the gut flora, but what this means in terms of changes in the gut lining, gut function, or gut symptoms is unclear. Whether menopause-related hormone treatments cause changes to the gut microbiota also remains unknown.

If you have had a hysterectomy (removal of the uterus due to fibroids or cancer), you may experience posthysterectomy gastrointestinal complications like fecal incontinence, although it's not entirely clear why.

seniors

Many chronic GI conditions affecting people
later in life, like cancer and cirrhosis, are
becoming increasingly common.

With life expectancy continuing to increase,
the elderly are the fastest-growing group in the
world. Some scientists hypothesize that parts
of the gut start to function less effectively
with age, although the evidence is not entirely
convincing. However, evidence is more
conclusive for higher rates of GERD and
constipation in this age group.

Dental and mouth issues

Dental issues become more common as we
age. Poor dental health and trauma from ill-
fitting dental prosthetics can have nutritional
consequences, with high rates of malnutrition
reported among older people. Also, changes in
taste can affect appetite and nutrient intake.
Neurologic conditions like stroke and Parkinson's
disease can also affect the ability to swallow.
A decrease in saliva production and an increase
in medications can cause dry mouth. Taking a
greater number of pills every day contributes to a
higher rate of "pill esophagitis" in older people,
where pills can get stuck in the esophagus and
cause inflammation. "Presbyesophagus" is a
loosely defined term describing changes in the
esophagus that come with advanced age that
put seniors at greater risk of developing pill
esophagitis, GERD, and motility disorders.

Medications

When seniors are prescribed more medications,
more gastrointestinal complications can occur.
Drug-induced liver injury may occur at higher
rates, especially as older people can suffer more
from mood and memory disorders that affect
their ability to take medications as advised. For
some, there is a higher risk of gastrointestinal
bleeding while taking blood thinners, which
are commonly prescribed for a variety of
cardiovascular conditions like atrial fibrillation
and cardiac stents after a heart attack. Higher
rates of cardiovascular disease can also affect
the gut. Mesenteric ischemia is a condition more
commonly seen in older individuals where the
gut circulation is compromised as the arteries
supplying the intestines can become clogged.

Constipation and gut motility

Constipation increases with age, with more
medications (like narcotic pain medications
and calcium channel blockers), other concurrent
conditions (like hypothyroidism), reduced
mobility, and a slowing of intestinal function.
Long-standing constipation over time also
predisposes the elderly to diverticular disease
in the colon, which can be complicated by

diverticulitis or diverticular bleeding. Due to reduced pelvic muscle function and rectal sensation, fecal incontinence is also more common among elderly patients. Fecal incontinence can be divided into three types: passive incontinence (unintentional passage of stool or gas), urge incontinence (passage despite attempts to retain fecal matter), and fecal seepage (following normal defecation).

Infections

As we age, we are more vulnerable to *Clostridioides difficile* infection, a diarrheal disease that can occur after a course of antibiotics, often associated with hospitals and nursing facilities. Compared to younger individuals, hospitalization rates are particularly high in the elderly (fourfold above age 65 and tenfold above age 85).

Cancer

Colorectal cancer rates are higher as age increases, with the median age of diagnosis at 66 years in men and 69 years in women. Fortunately, in recent years, we have seen rates of diagnosis and death at their lowest in history compared to previous decades in the US. Screening for colorectal cancer is typically recommended until age 75, although for healthy individuals above 75, screening may still be recommended for years thereafter. While the risk of colorectal cancer increases as we get older, the number of colorectal cancer diagnoses and deaths has fallen over the years, thanks to screening practices that allow for earlier detection and treatment.

COLORECTAL CANCER INCIDENT RATES BY AGE (US, 2012–2016)

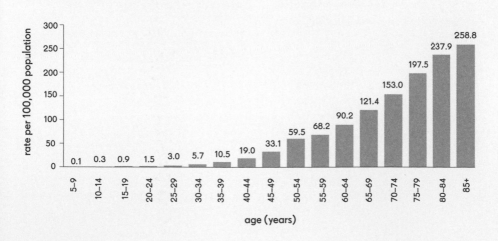

lifestyle check-in

For the best chance at maintaining good gut health,
take a moment to think about your diet and lifestyle,
and any changes you could make.

 ## Diet

• Aim for a balanced and diverse whole foods
diet to ensure you get all the macronutrients
and micronutrients needed for good gut
function. Your health-care system will provide
lots of free information to help guide you.

• Everything in moderation! If eaten infrequently
and in small amounts, occasional foods such as
red meat, cakes, and candy can still be part of
your diet.

• If you have a specific gut condition (like IBS
or celiac disease) or a goal in mind (like weight
loss), it may be best to talk with a dietitian to
agree on a tailored plan.

• Vitamin or mineral supplementation may be
recommended for some groups, and your GP
can request tests for you to ensure you have
adequate levels.

 ## Alcohol, smoking, recreational drugs

• Drinking alcohol and smoking not only cause
harm to organs like the esophagus, stomach,
and liver but may also increase your risk of
developing certain cancers of the gut or make
worse symptoms from existing conditions such
as Crohn's disease or chronic pancreatitis.

• Cocaine may reduce blood flow to the gut,
causing the bowel tissue to die (aka "ischemia").

• E-cigarettes or vaping may generate chemical
components that affect the gut barrier and
cause inflammation.

Hydration

- Drinking plain water is the best way to stay hydrated. However, consuming fruits and vegetables can help contribute to your daily fluid intake. Try vegetable juices and soups, green salads, and fruit and herbal teas. Drinking too many sugary or caffeinated drinks may leave you more dehydrated than when you started.

- Sometimes eight glasses of water aren't enough. The US National Academies of Sciences, Engineering, and Medicine recommends 11.5 to 15.5 glasses of water (92 to 124 fl oz / 2.6 to 3.6L) a day, and people who sweat more or are breastfeeding may require more.

 ## Sleep

- Variations in sleep schedules may impact the gut microbiota, potentially reducing microbial diversity and triggering changes in the immune system.

- Emerging research in 2023 found that even a 90-minute difference in sleep on weekdays versus weekends resulted in changes in the gut microbiota. However, some of this effect may be due to altered dietary choices and changes in appetite.

- Vice versa, some alterations in gut microbiota composition may also influence your circadian rhythm and sleep quality.

 ## Physical activity

- Remaining physically active not only helps with gut motility, but it may also help support your gut microbiota (see p.70).

 ## Home testing kits

- Several at-home testing kits are reported to detect a variety of conditions, including food allergies and sensitivities, with a finger prick, while others describe the gut microbiota composition in a stool sample. No home tests of this nature are FDA-approved, and many professional societies recommend against these tests due to potential inaccuracies and false positive tests, leading users to believe they may have certain conditions when they do not.

- Some at-home colorectal cancer screening tests are recommended. These tests help detect blood in stool and/or cancer-related DNA. While these kits can be convenient, there are still limitations to opting for noninvasive at-home tests. For instance, precancerous growths cannot be accurately located and removed at the time of diagnosis, which would be possible with a colonoscopy (see pp.138-139).

Q: SHOULD I ADOPT THE "CLEAN EATING" TREND?

A: While some people may interpret this dietary approach to mean avoiding ultra-processed food, others may focus on excluding certain food groups like starchy foods or consuming raw foods only. Cutting entire food groups out of one's diet is almost never recommended, as it can potentially limit access to important nutrients.

———

Q: ARE ALL PROCESSED FOODS BAD?

A: Anything that isn't straight off the farm is processed to some degree. Processed foods are not universally bad. In fact, some are deliberately fortified to meet certain nutritional needs. Freezing fruits and vegetables soon after harvesting can retain certain nutrients, unlike fresh produce that can spends days in transit before arriving in-store.

———

Q: IS ENDOSCOPY SAFE IN PREGNANCY?

A: The benefits of any procedure must be weighed up against its potential risks. Upper endoscopy and colonoscopy are safe during pregnancy if medically necessary. Addressing specific conditions like biliary gallstone disease may require special protocols to limit radiation exposure to the fetus.

———

Q: DOES HAVING A GUT ILLNESS AFFECT FERTILITY AND PREGNANCY OUTCOMES?

A: In patients with certain illnesses, like inflammatory bowel disease and celiac disease, there is some evidence showing higher rates of infertility, miscarriages, and preterm births. However, there is no clear mechanism to explain why patients are at higher risk of these events. Conversely, there have been reports of remission of some diseases during pregnancy for unknown reasons as well.

———

Q: SHOULD I AVOID ANTIBIOTICS?

A: Not if you need them! Keep in mind that antibiotics are used to prevent and treat certain bacterial infections. Antibiotics are not appropriate for viral infections like those associated with the common cold. If you are prescribed antibiotics for a bacterial infection, you should complete the entire course, even if you're feeling better. By ensuring the infection is fully dealt with before stopping antibiotics, there's less chance for resistance to develop.

———

Q: IS INTERMITTENT FASTING A GOOD WAY TO LOSE WEIGHT?

A: Experts often say that the best weight loss plan is the one that is sustainable. While some studies suggest that there are weight loss benefits and specifically fat loss benefits with intermittent fasting, the evidence remains unclear. There are many different patterns of fasting (time-restricted fasting during parts of the day versus alternate-day fasting, for instance), and there are no clear benefits of one strategy over another. Keep in mind that restricting eating to certain times does not equate to a free pass to eat less healthy foods or to binge eat.

———

Q: DO I NEED TO TAKE SUPPLEMENTS?

A: It's better to focus on improving the quality of your diet. Supplements are not a replacement for eating a balanced whole foods diet. However, for certain groups—pregnant women, kids, seniors, people with chronic conditions such as IBD, vegans—supplementation can be a necessary and helpful dietary addition.

———

Q: DOES ASPARTAME CAUSE CANCER?

A: In 2023, the World Health Organization's International Agency for Research on Cancer recategorized aspartame as a "possible carcinogen." However, this led to a debate among some experts since the WHO included, alongside aspartame, commonplace items like aloe vera and pickled vegetables.

———

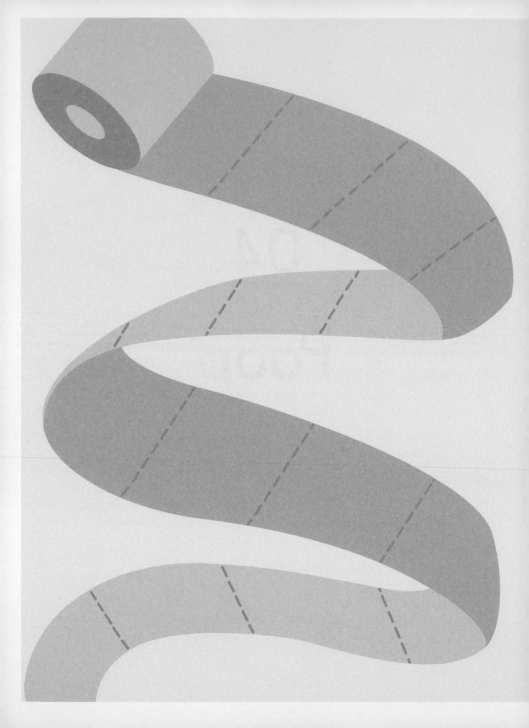

04

Poop

everybody poops

Whether you call it poop, poo, turd, stool, feces, or a number two, the need to produce excrement is universal!

Every day, there are approximately 352 fl oz (10 liters) of ingested food, fluid, and secretions, including saliva, gastric secretions, bile, and pancreatic juices, that travel through your gut. Water is mostly absorbed in the small intestine, although absorption starts in the stomach, but to a lesser extent. Poop is what is left over after food and liquid have passed through the gut, and water has been absorbed. By this point, 211 fl oz (6 liters) of water would have been extracted in the jejunum, and another 88 fl oz (2.5 liters) in the ileum, leaving around 53 fl oz (1.5 liters) on entering the colon. There, another 49 fl oz (1.4 liters) are absorbed, leaving 4 fl oz (0.1 liters) of water to be excreted.

Food processing

It takes approximately 10 to 70 hours for food to travel through the gut. Food consistency (solid or liquid), exercise, stress, medications, and some medical conditions can affect the length of time it takes for food to pass through the gut.

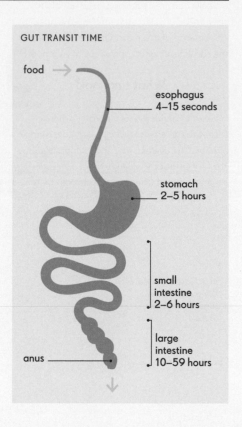

GUT TRANSIT TIME

food →

esophagus
4–15 seconds

stomach
2–5 hours

small
intestine
2–6 hours

large
intestine
10–59 hours

anus

What's in a turd?

Studies have shown that more than 50 percent of our poop is made up of water, with bacteria forming 25–54 percent of the dry component. Undigested fiber, carbohydrate, protein, fat, old cells from the gut lining, dead red blood cells, and mucus account for the remainder. The balance of these components can affect the consistency and appearance of your poo.

What's normal?

It's hard to define what is "normal" when it comes to the amount, weight, and consistency of poop. The average weight of a poop is about 7oz (200g), but this changes with diet, especially a high-fiber diet where more water can be mixed in with the stool. Even with a normal stool, there can be changes in consistency, color, and frequency that can determine whether it's "normal." Consistency of stool is not determined by what's in the stool, but on how fast poop travels through the colon. The longer it takes, the more water can be absorbed, leading to hard stools. Conversely, poop that travels rapidly through the gut retains a lot of water and comes out looser and more watery.

What about poop position?

The key to evacuating your bowel effectively is having your knees up higher than your hips—no easy thing when using a standard toilet, so a foot stool may help. In many societies, squatting is common, and some studies have shown that this position helps make pooping easier.

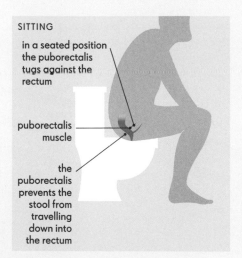

SITTING

in a seated position the puborectalis tugs against the rectum

puborectalis muscle

the puborectalis prevents the stool from travelling down into the rectum

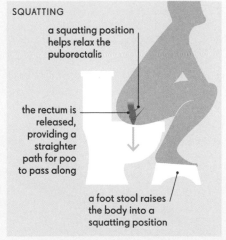

SQUATTING

a squatting position helps relax the puborectalis

the rectum is released, providing a straighter path for poo to pass along

a foot stool raises the body into a squatting position

the poop rainbow

The color of your poop can change depending on many factors, including what you eat or drink—think beets, a veggie that will give your poop a reddish hue.

 Brown

Poop is normally brown, mostly due to bile produced by your liver. Bile is typically an olive-green color when it is secreted into the intestine to help digest fats. A substance in bile called bilirubin, which is made up of old red blood cells, gets processed by the gut bacteria into stercobilin (a brown pigment). When mixed with undigested material, olive-green bile and processed bilirubin gives poop its characteristic brown color. Usually, poop remains a shade of brown, but there are some unusual situations that can influence the color of your poop.

 Red

Most commonly, red poop is a sign that there is fresh blood in your stool (known as hematochezia) coming from somewhere close to the anus as opposed to from the upper part of your gut like the stomach. Inflammation, trauma or fissures, bleeding vessels or other bleeding lesions (even tumors) can all cause red poop. The amount of blood may reveal the underlying cause. Small amounts of blood can stain an entire toilet bowl red, giving the appearance of far more blood than is actually there. Large amounts of blood don't necessarily spell danger, and not all red poop is caused by blood. The cause could be something as harmless as beets!

Black

Digested blood can form black poop, or "tarry stools." Bleeding in the upper digestive tract can be caused by stomach ulcers, small bowel lesions, or even a nosebleed. Iron supplements and bismuth salicylate found in antacids used to treat stomach and intestinal upsets are also common causes of black-colored poop.

Green

Green poop is often seen in people who eat lots of green, leafy vegetables. However, some conditions can result in green stools. The bacteria *Clostridioides difficile* causes watery, greenish diarrhea. Sometimes the antibiotics used to treat various infections can kill off the gut bacteria that help give poop its brown color, leaving the stool looking greener.

Yellow

Reduced production of bile can cause your poop to look more yellow. Stress, caffeine, and some medications can speed up intestinal movement, meaning less time for bile to be combined to give your poop its typical brown color. Also, when greater quantities of fats are consumed or when fat digestion is impaired, poop can appear more yellow, greasy, or fatty.

Gray

An obstruction to the normal flow of bile into the intestine can lead to gray or even white stools that resemble clay. An aggressive tumor can block the flow of bile, preventing it from coloring the stool, and if there is simultaneous upper gastrointestinal bleeding, the resulting black tarry mixture can give the stool a shiny silver appearance.

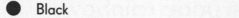

one lump or two

Firm, soft, or anywhere in between is considered
normal poop consistency. If your poop is too loose
or too hard, then something may have gone awry.

What makes your poop more solid or loose
depends on its physical makeup (how much
water-insoluble solids, such as fiber, electrolytes,
and dietary sugar are present) and the muscle
movement of your gut. Some medications
affect intestinal muscle movement, which can
in turn change the consistency of your poop.

In the foods we eat, there are two kinds of
fiber—soluble and insoluble—and the
consistency of your poop depends on the
balance between the two. Soluble fiber dissolves
in water, hydrating the stool into a gel-like
consistency. Insoluble fiber bulks up the stool so
that the gut can push it along more easily. While
there is no exact water-to-fiber ratio, too much
fiber without enough water will cause
constipation. Whereas too much water without
enough fiber may cause diarrhea.

Electrolyte imbalances in the gut can lead to
changes in stool consistency. Poorly absorbed
sugars, sugar alcohols, magnesium, sulfate, and
phosphate can cause stools to become loose.
Sugars that aren't fully absorbed across the
intestinal lining, including sucrose and lactose,
can cause loose stools in some people. This
sometimes becomes more apparent with age as
the enzyme that processes lactose, a sugar
found in milk, can disappear over time. Also,
certain disorders may change stool composition

leading to changes in consistency. For example,
disorders that limit a person's ability to digest
fats (see p140 and p148) can cause stools to
become oily and greasy.

Day-to-day differences in what we eat or
drink can directly affect the consistency of
our stool so a transient change is often normal.
Sustained changes in stool consistency, on
the other hand, should not be ignored. Change
in bowel habit should be reported to your
doctor for investigation.

Lastly, consistency of poop isn't all about
its composition. The speed of gut movement,
or transit time (see p88), will affect how much
water is absorbed. If things are moving fast,
diarrhea may result.

Stool type can indicate a patient may be
suffering from constipation, diarrhea, or even
a digestive condition, such as irritable bowel
syndrome (IBS). Stools should be soft and easy
to pass. To offer the best advice and treatment
plan, it's important for doctors to know what
a patient means by "loose stools."

BRISTOL STOOL CHART

Developed at the Bristol Royal Infirmary in 1997, the Bristol Stool Chart is used as a research tool to objectively describe stool consistency. The chart lists seven types of stools, which are different in shape, size, and consistency. Types 3 and 4 are considered "normal."

TYPE 1		Separate hard lumps that are difficult to pass
TYPE 2		Sausage shaped but lumpy
TYPE 3		Like a sausage but with cracks on the surface
TYPE 4		Like a sausage, smooth and soft
TYPE 5		Soft blobs with clear-cut edges (passed easily)
TYPE 6		Fluffy pieces with uneven edges
TYPE 7		No solid pieces, entirely liquid

all about gas

Whether it's the smell, the noise, or the bloating, gas
(or wind) can cause physical discomfort and embarrassment.
Let's explore everything you ever wanted to know about gas!

What's in a fart?

If you want to sound like an expert, the technical word for farting is flatulence. Researchers estimate there is 3.5–7 fl oz (100–200 ml) of gas in the intestines of a fasting person. Most people pass gas at least once a day and sometimes up to 20 times a day, although the number can vary with diet. About 90 percent of gas is comprised of nitrogen, oxygen, carbon dioxide, hydrogen, and methane.

Most gas resides in the colon. Gut bacteria produce gas when food is pushed from the small intestine into the colon. Most of these gases are odorless. The smelliness of a fart comes from very small amounts of hydrogen sulfide and methanethiol. Another interesting fact is that the gassiness felt after eating is not the direct result of fermented food, as much as it is gas being pushed downstream from the small intestine into the colon.

Where does gas come from and where does it go?

Gas can come from swallowing air, say when you're eating and talking, chemical reactions from food and medications, or from bacterial fermentation (like making kombucha in your

guts!). Carbohydrates like oats, potatoes, and corn are not fully absorbed by the small intestine, and when undigested food passes into the colon, gas is produced by bacteria in the gut. Sugars and sugar alcohols also contribute to gas production. Lactose in dairy products, fructose in fruit juice, and sugar alcohols, such as xylitol and sorbitol, used in chewing gum, are poorly absorbed and, when processed by bacteria in the gut, produce more gas.

Not all gas comes out of your rear, some of it comes out from your mouth as burps, while the rest is consumed by gut bacteria or absorbed into the blood.

COMPOSITION OF AN AVERAGE HUMAN FART

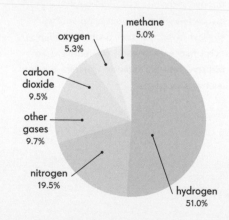

methane
5.0%

oxygen
5.3%

carbon
dioxide
9.5%

other
gases
9.7%

nitrogen
19.5%

hydrogen
51.0%

How does a fart happen?

When you fart, the body increases the pressure in the abdominal cavity and relaxes the anus to release gas. If there are any issues with muscle function and this sequence of events due to conditions like pelvic floor dyssynergia, it may be more difficult to pass gas. Lack of muscle coordination can cause poop and gas to be trapped in the intestines, which can bring discomfort and make your poop and gas smellier. In this situation, treatments such as pelvic floor exercises and biofeedback (see p181) are available to retrain muscles to help release trapped gas.

Fixing "abnormal" farts

Many patients ask me if they are passing too much gas, or why their farts smell so bad. The amount of farting can vary daily depending on what foods are eaten. Similarly, the smell of farts can be influenced by food choices and can be a sign of a microbial imbalance (excess of bacteria that produce sulfate and methane.) Foods rich in sulfur-containing compounds, like brassicas and onions, can cause stinkier farts, as can a diet high in animal proteins. These foods feed certain bacteria that produce smellier gas. However, if excess gas production is being caused by an underlying health condition, such as air-swallowing or lactose intolerance, caused by carbohydrate malabsorption, then this would need to be addressed first.

The good news is that in most cases the quantity and smell of farts can be altered by a change of diet. Foods that tend to increase gas production include beans, dairy products, some vegetables, and whole grains. Keeping a food diary may help identify trigger foods. Enzyme-based supplements containing alpha-galactosidase are used to reduce gas by helping break down certain carbohydrates, but the evidence is unclear as to their effectiveness.

The benefit of prebiotic or probiotic food or supplements is also unclear. Anecdotal evidence suggests that some people may find improvement in gas-related symptoms, while others find these supplements make their symptoms worse. If there is an underlying condition, like small intestine bacterial overgrowth (SIBO), antibiotics may be helpful.

Q: WHAT'S THE BEST FRUIT TO HELP RELIEVE CONSTIPATION?

A: There's not one fruit in particular that can help. It's best to eat a variety of fruits every week, especially high-fiber varieties like prunes and kiwi fruit, which support colonic contractions. Also try eating apples as they contain pectin, a fiber that turns into a gel that, when combined with water, helps ease constipation.

—

Q: HOW MANY TIMES SHOULD I POOP A DAY?

A: Everyone poops at a different pace! Just because you don't go every day doesn't necessarily mean there's something wrong with you. In fact, "normal" can be anywhere between three times a day and three times a week!

—

Q: I AM REGULARLY CONSTIPATED. DOES THIS MATTER?

A: Yes, as long-standing constipation can lead to problems such as hemorrhoids, anal fissures, and other gastrointestinal issues.

—

Q: IS POOPING A GOOD WAY TO LOSE WEIGHT?

A: Pooping more isn't going to lead to sustained weight loss. Therefore, stimulating bowel movements with laxatives isn't an effective (or healthy) way to lose weight.

—

Q: WHAT'S THE NAME FOR TOILET PHOBIA?

A: Parcopresis or "shy bowel syndrome" is the fear of or difficulty in having a poop in a public toilet.

—

Q: WHY DOES POOP FLOAT?

A: The composition of poop can vary depending on what is eaten: excess gas or fat in a stool can cause it to float. A change in your poop's buoyancy isn't in itself a cause for alarm.

—

Q: IS COLONIC HYDROTHERAPY SAFE?

A: Colonic hydrotherapy or colonic irrigation involves water being pumped through a tube into the colon via the anus. As the colon is hardwired to clean itself, there is no proven benefit that additional cleaning is beneficial, and it may cause harm. Mishandling of the tube can lead to bowel perforation, and infusing large amounts of water may cause electrolyte imbalances.

—

Q: CAN POOP BE USED AS FERTILIZER?

A: No, using human poop as fertilizer poses health risks as poop carries pathogens that can be transmitted between humans. Although there are strict sewage processes in place, these may not be sufficient in removing all harmful substances such as transmissible diseases or heavy metals.

—

Q: CAN GUT DEODORANTS HELP MAKE FARTS SMELL NICER?

A: Some products that include bismuth subgallate are marketed as gut deodorizers. While there may be some effect, there is no clear evidence of efficacy, and there have been reports of complications with long-term use.

—

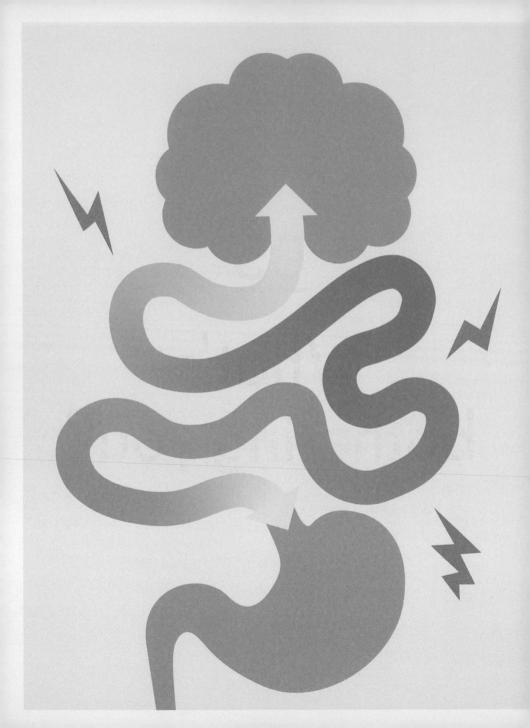

05

What's bothering you?

how are you feeling?

We often aren't really aware of our gut until something feels wrong. Let's look at the most common gut symptoms, and what they could mean for you.

Symptoms vary from person to person. Two individuals can experience one symptom differently—in severity, duration, and frequency. Triggers differ too. Some people never experience chronic illness, whereas others suffer from the same conditions for years, which can affect how symptoms are perceived. Even with the same illness, the pain might be severe for one person and mild for another. Sometimes a symptom appears in a subtle and insidious way, other times it is sudden and unexpected. Even a terminal illness like metastatic cancer can be diagnosed in someone with no symptoms at all.

If you're feeling under the weather, it can be tempting to turn to Doctor Google. But this isn't always the best source of relevant medical information. You know what's normal for your body, and you will usually be able to feel when something isn't quite right. If you've spoken to your pharmacist and over-the-counter medications aren't helping, book an appointment with your doctor.

Let's take a look at 10 of the most common symptoms you may experience in your everyday life— these are symptoms your doctor will regularly encounter. Let's look at each symptom in turn, and see how your doctor might diagnose your condition, and then what treatment you might be offered, if needed.

If you're feeling under the weather, it can be tempting to turn to Doctor Google.

SYMPTOM ASSESSMENT

"OPQRST" is a mnemonic used by doctors for patient assessment. Typically used to evaluate pain, this approach can be applied to other symptoms, too. OPQRST stands for onset, provocation (or palliation), quality, region (or radiation), severity, and time.

	ONSET	When did your symptom begin? Did it start suddenly or come on gradually? Was there a trigger for this symptom?
	PROVOCATION/ PALLIATION	Does anything make the symptom better or worse? If you tried treating it, what seemed to help, or what made it worse?
	QUALITY	Describe your pain—is it sharp, burning, achy, throbbing? What color and consistency is your stool?
	REGION	Where is the pain located? Does it stay in the same area, or does it tend to move around?
	SEVERITY	Is the pain mild, moderate, or severe? How bad is it on a scale of 1 to 10, with 10 being the worst? For bleeding, is it a large or a small amount?
	TIME	How long ago did the symptom start, e.g., recently (acute) or has it been going on for a while (chronic)? Does it come and go, or is it constant?

jaundice

Jaundice is a yellowing of parts
of your body due to increased levels of
a yellow pigment, bilirubin, in the blood.

Symptoms Jaundice is when there is yellowing of the skin, eyes, and mucous membranes. Bilirubin is mainly produced during the breakdown of red blood cells; if there is a buildup of bilirubin—for instance, as a result of conditions like liver cirrhosis where there is scarring and dysfunction in the liver—this can result in jaundice. Jaundice can also represent problems with the gallbladder, or bile ducts where a disorder in the production or transport of bile can develop. Cholestasis (slow-flowing bile) in pregnancy can lead to jaundice, but it eventually clears after delivery. Jaundice can also occur when a gallstone gets lodged in the bile duct and the bile is unable to empty into the intestine. If bilirubin builds up to a high enough level, patients may experience itchiness as another symptom.

Diagnosis In addition to a medical history, blood tests will confirm if the yellow discoloration is due to a bilirubin issue and the result of a specific underlying condition. For structural problems like a gallstone or tumor blocking the bile duct, a CT scan or MRI may reveal the underlying issue. If liver disease is suspected, a liver biopsy may be necessary to look for microscopic abnormalities.

Treatment If jaundice is the result of a mechanical obstruction, endoscopic procedures may be required to relieve the blockage, including removing gallstones lodged in the bile duct or placing a stent to open a bile duct blocked by an encroaching tumor. Failure to relieve a blockage can quickly become a serious problem because stagnant bile can easily become infected. Should a resectable (operable) cancer be found, then surgery may be required for a long-term solution. When jaundice is not caused by a blockage, but rather by some other underlying disease, certain medications such as ursodeoxycholic acid can help clear the jaundice. Avoiding toxins like alcohol may also be recommended to prevent further damage to the liver. Even in rapidly reversible conditions, jaundice and the associated itchiness can take days to weeks to clear up.

Jaundice can also represent problems with the gallbladder, or bile ducts.

dysphagia

Dysphagia is the medical term for having difficulty when swallowing either solid food or liquid.

Symptoms Dysphagia can occur during the active phase of swallowing. To doctors, "swallowing" refers to both the active motion of pushing food down the back of the throat, but also the automatic movement of the esophagus pushing food down into the stomach. Dysphagia can be a result of neuromuscular disorders like Parkinson's disease, or a physical obstruction from a tumor or spinal bony protrusion. Movement disorders of the esophagus such as achalasia (where the sphincter between the esophagus and stomach will not relax) can cause dysphagia. Inflammatory conditions like eosinophilic esophagitis can lead to difficulty swallowing as can injury to the esophagus due to acid reflux.

Pain experienced when swallowing is called odynophagia. A sore throat can be caused by an infection and inflammation of the esophagus lining, as is the case with strep throat, or the tonsils (in tonsillitis). Ulcers, tumors, or lodged foreign objects like fish bones can lead to discomfort when swallowing, too.

Diagnosis Disorders of swallowing can be diagnosed by ruling out any mechanical obstruction using an X-ray (barium swallow) and/or an endoscopy. The contractility and muscle function of the esophagus can be evaluated using a medical tool called esophageal manometry. Other procedures like pH testing may be required to assess for associated conditions like acid reflux.

Treatment The underlying cause will determine the recommended treatment. Adjusting food choices, food consistency, and eating habits are the usual first steps to relieving symptoms. Oral medication can help with esophageal muscle movement, and surgical procedures may provide relief, too. For achalasia, the muscle that will not relax at the bottom of the esophagus can be cut either surgically (Heller myotomy) or endoscopically through the mouth (peroral endoscopic myotomy, or POEM for short). For odynophagia, there are topical medications and lozenges that can help relieve discomfort.

heartburn

The burning sensation felt in the chest is typically related
to gastroesophageal reflux when stomach juices
frequently travels up into the esophagus.

Symptoms Pain is often felt at the bottom of the breastbone, which is where the esophagus is connected to the stomach. This sensation can become worse when lying down. Sometimes the acid that is regurgitated can travel all the way up the esophagus and cause other symptoms like a chronic cough or vocal changes related to irritation of the airway.

Everyone experiences acid reflux—it's a normal phenomenon—but if you are experiencing more severe symptoms such as having difficulty swallowing, and if over-the-counter medication is not helping, you might want to seek medical attention. What makes gastroesophageal reflux (GERD) become a *disorder* is an unusual amount of reflux due to a weak or overly relaxed lower esophageal sphincter. There is limited evidence to prove that certain foods cause increased acid reflux, although there are many anecdotal triggers, including citrus fruits, spicy foods, caffeine, and chocolate. Some patients with GERD might not experience any heartburn at all. You might experience GERD as a side effect of certain medications.

Risk factors include central (abdominal) obesity or pregnancy due to increased intra-abdominal pressure that pushes acid up in the wrong direction, and also the presence of a hiatus hernia where part of the stomach protrudes into the chest. Although GERD is rarely deadly, it poses a significant burden on the health system from its complications, like esophageal inflammation, strictures, and Barrett's esophagus (precancerous changes from long-standing acid exposure to the esophagus).

Diagnosis When GERD is suspected, a trial of medication is often recommended. Additional testing may be required to confirm the diagnosis if symptoms remain. These tests may include pH monitoring to measure the pH of the esophagus, an endoscopy to visualize any acid injury or structural defects, or performing biopsies in the affected areas to rule out Barrett's esophagus. Note that GERD is not specific to acid reflux. Nonacid reflux is also a phenomenon that may result in the same symptoms.

Treatment A trial of proton pump inhibitor (PPI) medications to suppress acid is often the first-line treatment. Histamine blockers and antacids are also commonly prescribed. Lifestyle modifications, such as avoiding dietary triggers, sitting upright, eating smaller meals, adjusting your pillows to elevate your head when sleeping, and weight loss for those who may have increased central obesity can be helpful. If symptoms remain uncontrolled on medicine, or long-term medication is required, patients may be referred for an endoscopic or surgical anti-reflux procedure. This procedure is called fundoplication and involves wrapping the upper portion of the stomach around the bottom of the esophagus to restore the barrier and prevent acid from traveling back up into the esophagus.

LOOSE ESOPHAGUS

One of the consequences of long-standing acid exposure to the esophagus as a result of GERD is Barrett's esophagus. The associated changes to the esophagus lining can potentially turn cancerous over time. Controlling acid production with medication can help prevent these cellular changes from occurring. If precancerous changes are found, they can potentially be treated to prevent esophageal cancer from occurring (see p126).

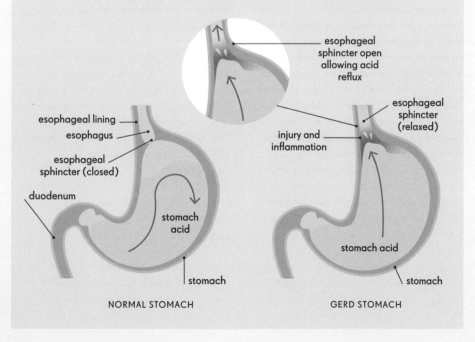

esophageal sphincter open allowing acid reflux

esophageal sphincter (relaxed)

esophageal lining

esophagus

injury and inflammation

esophageal sphincter (closed)

duodenum

stomach acid

stomach acid

stomach

stomach

NORMAL STOMACH

GERD STOMACH

loss of appetite and weight loss

Although appetite can fluctuate day to day, prolonged loss
of appetite can signify something more serious.

Symptoms If you are losing weight and don't know why (for instance, if your appetite and food consumption remain the same and you are still losing weight), it can be alarming. As these symptoms are not specific to one condition, a thorough medical history and physical examination are important to uncover the underlying condition, or medication side effects. Unintentional weight loss can be caused by a number of conditions, such as anxiety and depression, IBD (see pp136–138), IBS (see pp133–134), or celiac disease (see pp135–136), although sometimes other more likely symptoms like diarrhea are the cause.

Diagnosis Understanding the eating habits and dietary patterns of patients can be helpful in identifying a cause. Medications often impact appetite, so learning when symptoms began is key. Loss of appetite can be caused by certain medications, poor dental hygiene or oral lesions, an altered sense of taste and smell, or chronic nausea or vomiting that is triggered by eating.

While the underlying causes of loss of appetite can be a physical medical condition, there are other mental health disorders that can severely impact appetite and weight loss. A doctor should carefully assess for disordered eating and make sure that appropriate psychiatric referrals for support are made if necessary.

Your doctor may carry out blood tests to rule out certain cancers or nutritional deficiencies (see p50) or refer you for an X-ray to rule out any structural issues, such as tumors. Doctors must join together pieces of evidence to get a complete picture.

Treatment While treating the underlying cause is the most important factor in reversing the loss of appetite and weight loss, in some chronic diseases or incurable illnesses, long-term nutritional supplements may be required. Replenishing nutrition through oral supplementation or intravenously requires careful monitoring to avoid refeeding syndrome or the risk of infection. Appetite stimulants might also be considered, but there is little data to show any long-term survival benefit from using these stimulants.

• UNEXPLAINED WEIGHT LOSS •

The phrase "unintentional weight loss" can ring an alarm bell to a doctor as it may indicate a potential undiagnosed cancer. Some cancers are metabolically active and consume energy, which can lead to unintentional weight loss.

nausea and vomiting

All of us have experienced nausea or vomiting, or both,
so can relate to how unpleasant they are.

Symptoms Nausea is the sensation of discomfort in the stomach, often accompanied by an urge to vomit. Vomiting, on the other hand, is a forceful ejection through the mouth of stomach contents with contraction of the diaphragm and associated abdominal muscles. Regurgitation, unlike vomiting, is a different condition that describes a passive upward movement of content from the stomach into the esophagus that is not preceded by nausea.

Nausea and vomiting occur due to a vomiting center in the brain being triggered by signals from the gut. However, vomiting events can vary by time of day, meals consumed, odor and appearance of the vomited material, and whether strong retching and projectile vomiting occur. Some causes may be directly due to gut issues such as structural blockages, infection, or organs inflammation, while others include systemic disorders, medications, or substances that cause nausea and vomiting as side effects.

Diagnosis While blood tests may reveal underlying causes like infections, electrolyte imbalances, or other organ dysfunction, imaging and endoscopy may be necessary to assess for structural problems. A gastric emptying study can potentially identify any movement disorders of the stomach that can lead to the buildup of undigested food, resulting in vomiting.

> • NON-PHARMACOLOGICAL INTERVENTIONS •
>
> **Relaxation techniques** such as deep breathing exercises or meditation can help reduce nausea and promote relaxation. **Acupressure or acupuncture** can provide relief for some individuals.

Treatment Aside from addressing any underlying disease directly, medications may need to be stopped or adjusted. Anti-nausea medications or medications that promote gut motility may help alleviate symptoms for short-term conditions. In some cases, adjusting dietary habits and opting to eat small, frequent meals can help. With frequent vomiting, it is important to replenish fluids and electrolytes to prevent dehydration and more serious electrolyte imbalances. Persistent or severe nausea and vomiting that cannot be managed with over-the-counter remedies or lifestyle modifications should be evaluated by a health-care professional.

bloating and burping

Gas and bloating are common symptoms
that often go hand in hand, but the causes and
treatments are not always straightforward.

Symptoms Bloating refers to a gassy
sensation of fullness in the abdomen and
visible distension (belly swelling), although
not everyone experiences belly swelling when
bloated. Gas in the digestive system is primarily
produced from swallowing air or from the
breakdown of food during digestion. Some
foods may be more prone to causing gas than
others (see pp94–95). Underlying
gastrointestinal disorders like IBS or lactose
intolerance can increase gas and bloating. Some
people may be more sensitive or respond
differently to gas buildup compared to others.
Similarly, how intestinal muscles or the
diaphragm respond to allow room for gassy
intestines can vary from person to person.

Burping or belching is a normal bodily
function to expel air out of the mouth.
Generally, a burp is air swallowed while eating
and drinking, especially while chewing gum,
and consuming carbonated drinks. For people
who think they burp more often than usual,
stress, psychiatric disorders, or the unconscious
swallowing of air may be the cause. Counseling
and breathing techniques can help in these
cases. Some people are unable to burp,
especially those with "gas-bloat syndrome,"
which can happen after fundoplication
surgery where the bottom of the esophagus
is tightened to prevent acid reflux. Stinky
burps can be a sign of other diseases like
gastroparesis where the food lingers in the

• "HOW TO GET RID OF
BLOATING, FAST" •

There are lots of myths around bloating
such as drinking coffee or celery juice but
some bloating is completely normal, and
will go away on its own. If you experience
chronic, uncomfortable bloating though, it
could be worth speaking to your doctor.

stomach for abnormally long periods due to slow stomach emptying. Bacteria in ear, sinus, or throat infections can also create smelly sulfur-containing gases. A patient with cirrhosis (liver disease) cannot remove certain toxins like ammonia, which then accumulate in the blood and are exhaled by the lungs, causing foul smelling breath called "fetor hepaticus". The smell is sometimes described as a combination of rotten eggs and garlic.

Diagnosis Blood tests and imaging studies, including X-rays, scans, or an endoscopy, can be helpful in identifying any underlying cause. For instance, a biopsy taken during an endoscopy may reveal findings that suggest celiac disease. Other tests include specific breath tests that measure certain gases that are released after drinking a sugary syrup. These tests may point toward conditions like small intestine bacterial overgrowth (SIBO), or intolerances to lactose or fructose. Testing is often unnecessary for lactose intolerance, and a presumed diagnosis can be made if there is a response to a lactose-free diet.

Treatment Where diet is a factor, identifying trigger foods may provide the solution, as is the case with lactose and lactose intolerance and gluten and celiac disease. For other disorders like IBS, following a low-FODMAP diet may help and involves eliminating certain foods high in FODMAPs and then later reintroducing them one by one to identify specific triggers. Adjusting eating habits, such as timing and frequency of meals, along with chewing food slowly to minimize air swallowing may also help. Some medications like antispasmodics may be prescribed to help manage the symptoms associated with bloating. Laxatives and antidiarrheals may also help those with associated constipation or diarrhea.

Burping or belching is a normal bodily function to expel air out of the mouth.

abdominal pain

Not all abdominal pain is the same; it often corresponds to specific areas of the abdomen and can have many different causes.

PAIN MAP

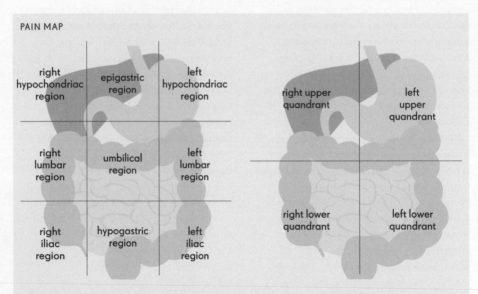

For the purpose of helping doctors identify the potential organ that's causing pain, the abdomen is divided into various parts. Characterizing the pain through further questioning, physical examination, and imaging can help guide doctors to the most likely diagnosis.

Symptoms Abdominal pain can vary from sharp, stabbing, and burning to achy and gassy, or all of these. The pain can be unrelenting or intermittent, local or systemic, and mild or severe. Abdominal pain can originate from any of the organs within the abdominal cavity, including the stomach, liver, gallbladder,

intestines, appendix, kidneys, and reproductive organs. As there are numerous causes for abdominal pain, doctors must piece together various characteristics and try to determine a diagnosis. It's important to get context by taking a thorough medical history to understand the events that led to the onset of pain, including any underlying medical problems, recent changes in medication, or other relevant experiences.

Diagnosis Doctors may use the "OPQRST" approach to characterize symptoms and help support a diagnosis. Other associated symptoms like fever, nausea, vomiting, or blood in the stool may also indicate a certain diagnosis. For example, acute pancreatitis is often described as acute, sharp epigastric pain that radiates to the back, with pain relieved by leaning forward and worsened when lying flat, and sometimes associated with nausea and vomiting.

A physical examination can help doctors further evaluate the pain by visually inspecting, listening, tapping, and pressing on the abdomen. For instance, seeing a distended abdomen and hearing a lack of bowel sounds may suggest ileus (the small intestine stops moving). Blood tests can help check for markers of inflammation or infection, and sometimes indicate which organ may be affected. To get a better look at those organs, imaging studies like ultrasound, X-rays, scans, and even an endoscopy can help doctors identify the source of pain.

Treatment The treatment of abdominal pain depends on the underlying cause. In some instances, simple measures can help alleviate symptoms. Conditions such as food poisoning can quickly resolve with rest and hydration; other conditions take time to improve and may need the help of medication. For example, gastroesophageal reflux disease (GERD)

gradually responds to acid-suppressing medication. Conditions such as acute pancreatitis or an IBD flare, may require hospitalization for closer monitoring and treatment. Others may even require emergency surgery to remove a diseased organ like an appendectomy for appendicitis. Over-the-counter pain relief can be helpful but some treatments, like nonsteroidal anti-inflammatory drugs (NSAIDs), can make worse some problems, such as stomach ulcers.

It is important to acknowledge that not all abdominal pain is caused by something structurally abnormal. The brain and gut are intimately linked, and emotional stress can augment the pain experienced. Just because there is not something detected on a scan doesn't make the pain imaginary or any less than what someone is reporting. Pain without a structural explanation can still be debilitating and significantly impact a person's quality of life. There may be symptom-directed treatments and behavioral therapies that could alleviate pain and restore some normalcy to an individual's life.

Abdominal pain can originate from any of the organs within the abdominal cavity.

constipation

Most people have experienced constipation,
but a chronic case may need treatment
beyond dietary changes.

Symptoms Constipation is a common symptom, described as having infrequent bowel movements or difficulty passing a poop. Most people who have constipation have it occasionally, without needing any treatment. Constipation can vary based on the frequency of bowel movements, how much straining is required, how firm the stool is, a feeling of incomplete emptying, a blockage, or the need to manually remove a poop.

Some causes of constipation are limited to the intestine itself, like constipation predominant chronic idiopathic constipation (CIC) and irritable bowel syndrome with constipation (IBS-C). CIC is thought to be due to the slow transit of a stool through the colon. The main difference between IBS-C and CIC is the presence of pain and discomfort in IBS-C. The cause of IBS-C is thought to be less about slow transit than as genetic, environmental, and psychological factors.

There can be other "secondary" causes of constipation, such as a mechanical blockage from scar tissue or a tumor that prevents passage of poop. Constipation can be a side effect of certain medical conditions, such as hypothyroidism, diabetes, and neurological disorders, including multiple sclerosis, stroke, or amyloidosis. Pregnancy may cause constipation due to hormonal changes that affect intestinal movement. Also, many medications, such as opioid pain medications, certain anti-depressants, iron supplements, and some antacids, can also slow intestinal movement.

Diagnosis Unless it is chronic or severe, many doctors diagnosing constipation do not go beyond asking some basic questions about frequency of bowel movement, poop consistency, and ruling out secondary causes of constipation. One simple test is a rectal examination, where the doctor inserts a gloved finger into the rectum to make sure there isn't something obvious like a tumor preventing stool from coming out. But if the constipation is still unexplained, doctors may choose to perform additional blood tests, imaging studies, and/or a colonoscopy to look for other underlying diseases or structural

Long-term use of any laxative should be evaluated by a professional.

problems that might be preventing the passing of a regular, smooth poop. There are also imaging studies that look specifically at how long it takes for a stool to travel through the colon. There are other tests to assess the squeezing ability of muscles involved in defecation (see p83). Rather than a problem with intestinal movement, it may be that the pelvic floor muscles lack coordination with the anal sphincter muscle when pushing out a poop.

Treatment Dietary adjustments are often considered a first-line approach in the prevention and treatment of constipation. With the right combination of fluid and fiber intake, stool consistency and regularity may improve. Staying physically active and reducing psychological stressors can also help promote intestinal movement and improve constipation.

There are a variety of medical therapies to treat constipation. One kind of medication is a stool softener, which lubricates the stool by drawing in more water or fat from the colon. Osmotic laxatives (like magnesium citrate) work by drawing fluid into the intestine, helping to soften poop. Stimulant laxatives (like senna) stimulate intestinal muscles to accelerate the speed of poop through the intestine. Some prescription-only medications (like lubiprostone, linaclotide, plecanatide, or prucalopride) can improve fluid secretion from the bowel lining and speed up intestinal transit and are used for specific conditions like IBS-C. Long-term use of any laxative should be evaluated by a professional. Some categories, like stimulant laxatives, may lead to dependency on the drug to pass a poop and may become less effective over time.

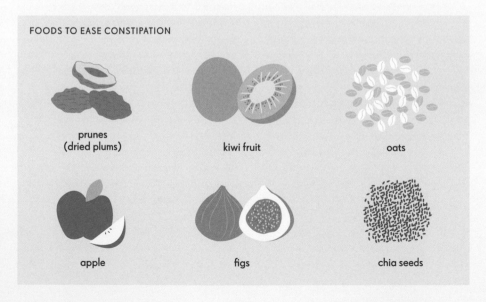

FOODS TO EASE CONSTIPATION

prunes
(dried plums)

kiwi fruit

oats

apple

figs

chia seeds

diarrhea

Everyone experiences diarrhea at least once
in their lifetime, and like constipation, it
is a symptom, not a disease itself.

Symptoms More than three bowel movements
a day would be considered unusual, although
the quantity and consistency of the stool can
still vary. Most cases of diarrhea can be put
into two main categories: osmotic or secretory.
These two types of diarrhea are not mutually
exclusive, and some conditions can lead to
both osmotic and secretory diarrhea.

Osmotic diarrhea is when too much water
is drawn into the gut by nutrients or molecules
in the gut. For instance, in patients who are
lactose intolerant, undigested lactose will draw
water into the intestine and lead to looser stools.
When these molecules are no longer ingested,
osmotic diarrhea goes away.

Secretory diarrhea is when something, often an
infection, stimulates cells in the intestine to
actively secrete electrolytes, attracting water as a
result. This also happens in conditions like
inflammatory bowel disease (IBD) and celiac
disease where damage to the intestinal lining
makes it harder for the intestine to absorb water.

Diagnosis For doctors, trying to figure out the
cause of diarrhea requires determining whether
it's an acute or chronic problem, if there's usually
a large or small volume of diarrhea passed,
and whether the diarrhea is watery, fatty, or
bloody in nature. Then, a doctor would want to
know whether there are any underlying medical
conditions, if the patient is using specific
medications, or has been traveling overseas.

Diarrhea that lasts less than four weeks is
considered acute diarrhea, with most causes
related to an infection or a new medication.
Whereas diarrhea that lasts more than four
weeks is categorized as chronic. Some causes
include malabsorption syndromes such as celiac
disease and lactose intolerance, or infections like
Clostridioides difficile, cytomegalovirus, and
herpes simplex virus. Other causes include
ischemic colitis, IBD, disordered motility
(diabetic neuropathy), IBS, or endocrine
disorders and tumors. There are also rare
situations of chronic diarrhea due to people
relying on enteral feeding (feeding tube) for their
nutrition. Figuring out what is causing diarrhea
may require stool studies, blood tests, scans,
and imaging tests such as a colonoscopy.

OSMOTIC VS. SECRETORY DIARRHEA

In a healthy gut, fluid leaves the intestinal lumen (cavity) and is absorbed by the body. But with osmotic or secretory diarrhea, there is a buildup of fluid within the intestine.

OSMOTIC

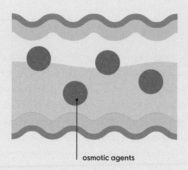

osmotic agents

SECRETORY

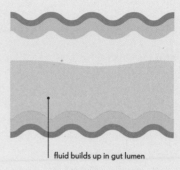

fluid builds up in gut lumen

In osmotic diarrhea, "osmotic agents", such as lactose or sucrose, attract fluid into the gut.

In secretory diarrhea, fluid builds up inside the gut cavity, drawn in by electrolytes secreted by cells in the intestine.

Treatment Different approaches may be taken depending on the underlying cause of the diarrhea. Since acute diarrhea is often associated with infections, an antibiotic is sometimes recommended. If the specific cause of infection is identified, a targeted antibiotic or antiparasitic therapy may be prescribed.

For chronic diarrhea, aside from treating the underlying condition, some doctors may recommend antidiarrheal agents to slow the movement of the gut for symptom relief.

Certain medications may be recommended to help remove excess bile following a cholecystectomy (gallbladder removal) that may cause diarrhea. To identify the cause, stools are collected and examined for inflammatory cells and specific bacteria, or measurements taken of electrolytes or fat content to help determine the underlying cause.

incontinence

Fecal incontinence is a distressing (and
often stigmatized) condition, which can be
uncomfortable and embarrassing.

Symptoms Fecal incontinence is characterized
by the leakage of stool, or inability to control
bowel movements. Incontinence can also be
inconvenient and costly to maintain personal
hygiene. In addition to the impact on quality
of life from the underlying medical condition,
incontinence can also result in constant fear of
accidents and lead to social isolation. There can
be several potential causes of fecal incontinence,
including muscle or nerve damage to the pelvic
floor muscles or around the anus because of
trauma, or neurological conditions like multiple
sclerosis. However, incontinence can also be due
to chronic diarrhea or constipation.

Diagnosis In addition to evaluating the severity
of the incontinence, doctors may choose to
perform various tests to discover where the
dysfunction lies. A rectal examination may be
required to assess the integrity of the sphincter
muscle and the squeezing ability of the rectum.
Certain blood and stool tests may be ordered to
check whether there is uncontrolled diabetes or
an underlying infectious disease.

To make sure there are no other concerning
issues, like a tumor causing a blockage and
overflowing of liquid stool, a colonoscopy may
be necessary to take a closer look inside the
rectum. Special endoscopes equipped with

ultrasound can help doctors assess the muscle
layers of the anus. Another imaging test is
defecography, where the rectum is filled with
barium paste and either an X-ray or MRI
machine will take pictures of the rectum while
the patient passes the paste. To measure
muscle function, anorectal manometry can be
performed to measure the squeezing pressures
in the rectum and anus. A balloon expulsion test
can also be done to see if those muscles can
actively push out an air- or water-filled balloon.

Treatment The treatment for fecal incontinence
depends on the underlying cause and severity
of the condition. In mild cases, dietary changes
such as increasing fiber intake to regulate bowel
movements may be adequate. In cases where
diarrhea is the underlying issue, medications like
antidiarrheals or fiber supplements can help
create firmer stools. Pelvic floor muscle exercises
such as Kegel exercises may also help
strengthen the muscles that control bowel
movements. Biofeedback therapy and
implantable nerve stimulators can help train
and strengthen the pelvic floor and anal
sphincter muscles. For more severe cases of
fecal incontinence, surgery may be considered
to repair the anal sphincter or insert an
artificial anal sphincter.

defecatory disorders

These disorders describe conditions where there are difficulties in evacuating stools, either due to muscle discoordination or structural issues with the rectum.

Symptoms Anorectal dysfunction is where the muscles and nerves around the anus do not function, which prevents the anus from opening and allowing stools to exit. Pelvic floor dyssynergia causes muscle discoordination that affects the muscles of the pelvic floor, preventing stools from passing.

A rectocele is a bulging of the wall of the rectum, which may make it difficult for the rectal muscles to push poop out normally. A rectal prolapse can cause difficulty in evacuating stools as weakness in the rectal muscles cause the rectum to protrude outside the body.

Diagnosis When a defecatory disorder is suspected, some tests that are performed include a defecography, balloon expulsion test, and anorectal manometry.

Defecography is when the rectum is filled with a radiopaque liquid and the patient is asked to strain while X-ray images are taken. For a balloon expulsion test, a balloon is inserted into the rectum and inflated, and the patient is then asked to push the balloon out while being timed.

Anorectal manometry involves a catheter being inserted into the rectum to measure the squeezing pressures of the anal and rectal muscles. Sometimes if the anal sphincter

squeezes are too tight relative to the rectal muscles during defecation, a diagnosis of dyssynergia might be suspected.

Treatment For defecatory disorders, there may be a need for specific training or biofeedback therapy to improve toilet behaviors and reset the muscle coordination between the rectum and anus. At times, more invasive therapies like Botox injections into the pelvic muscles or surgery to remove part of the colon may be required to provide relief for people who suffer from severe and persistent constipation.

For a balloon expulsion test, a balloon is inserted into the rectum and inflated.

Your questions answered

Q: IS A GASTRIC ULCER CAUSED BY STRESS ALONE?

A: No, increased smoking, drinking alcohol, and NSAID pain medication use can also increase the risk for gastric ulcers. As well as psychological stress, physiological stress (meaning, from a severe medical condition) can also increase the risk.

—

Q: WILL EATING SPICY OR FATTY FOODS MAKE MY REFLUX WORSE?

A: While the scientific data remains unclear, anecdotally, many people report that these foods can worsen their acid reflux. There are many potential triggers for acid reflux, so it's best to avoid what you know can bring about those symptoms.

—

Q: IS ALL ABDOMINAL PAIN AN EMERGENCY?

A: While there are certain causes of abdominal pain that require immediate intervention (like appendicitis), other causes of abdominal pain can often resolve on their own. Sometimes there are other associated symptoms, like fever, that point to a more serious condition. When in doubt, it's best to be evaluated in person by a professional.

—

Q: IS HAVING BLOOD IN YOUR POOP ALWAYS A SIGN OF COLON CANCER?

A: Blood in the stool is never "normal" in itself. For that reason, it is important to see a doctor to make sure serious causes like colon cancer are ruled out. Many "benign" conditions can also result in bleeding, including hemorrhoids, anal fissures, or bleeding colonic diverticula.

—

Q: DOES ALL ABDOMINAL PAIN COME FROM ORGANS?

No, the abdominal wall can also be a cause of pain. Sometimes muscle or nerve injury can lead to pain, but it's not from an organ within the abdominal cavity. Moreover, the inner wall of the abdominal cavity (peritoneum) can also be irritated or inflamed because of infected fluid in the abdomen, which can lead to pain.

Q: IS ACID REFLUX ALWAYS ACCOMPANIED BY HEARTBURN?

A: Not everyone with acid reflux presents with heartburn. Some people go about their day without any symptoms yet during an endoscopy are found to have signs of chronic inflammation related to acid reflux. Others have less typical symptoms like hoarseness and other vocal changes related to acid refluxing up the esophagus toward the airway where the vocal cords sit.

Q: ARE NAUSEA AND VOMITING ALWAYS THE RESULT OF A GUT PROBLEM?

A: Not necessarily. Some ear conditions can cause nausea and dizziness by disturbing how our bodies regulate balance. There are some brain disorders that can lead to intractable nausea and vomiting.

Q: IS VOMITING BLOOD EVER NORMAL?

A: No, vomiting blood is never normal. Sometimes vomiting after consuming a red-colored food or drink, like beet juice, can mimic blood, but if this isn't the case, please speak with your doctor.

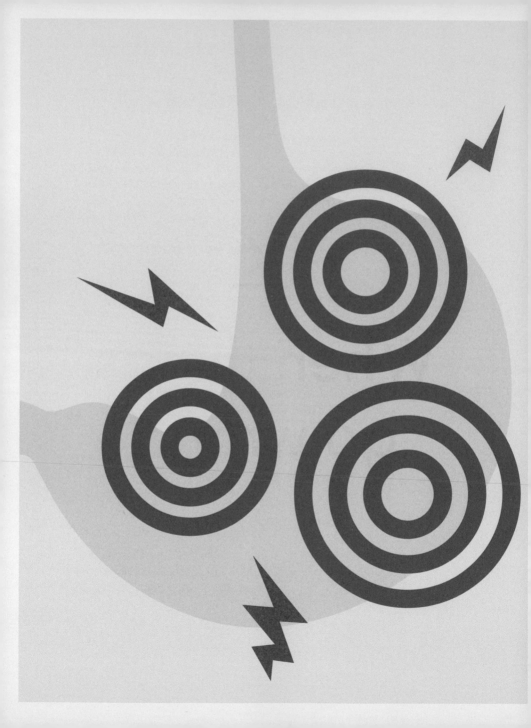

06

When things
go wrong

digestive disorders

A lot can go wrong with the gut, but no one person will
have all the conditions about to be discussed here.
Let's take a look from top to bottom.

THE GUT FROM TOP TO BOTTOM

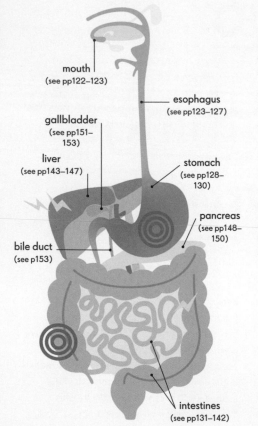

mouth
(see pp122–123)

gallbladder
(see pp151–
153)

liver
(see pp143–147)

bile duct
(see p153)

esophagus
(see pp123–127)

stomach
(see pp128–
130)

pancreas
(see pp148–
150)

intestines
(see pp131–142)

Mouth and esophagus

DRY MOUTH (XEROSTOMIA)

Dry mouth (xerostomia) is a condition where
the production of saliva is reduced, leading
to difficulty chewing, blunted taste and smell,
a sore throat, and a greater risk of developing
cavities. This can be caused by conditions that
affect the salivary glands, including radiotherapy,
autoimmune conditions such as Sjogren's
Syndrome, as well as certain anti-depressants,
blood pressure medications, antihistamines,
and more.

Diagnosis is often a "clinical diagnosis" based on
symptoms rather than tests, although specific
tests for underlying diseases may be requested.

Treatment depends on the cause and can be as
simple as changing implicated medications.

CANDIDIASIS (THRUSH)

Candidiasis (thrush) occurs in the oral cavity and presents as white plaques, typically caused by the fungal species *Candida*. *Candida* is normally present in the mouth but can overgrow, especially after steroid therapy or other scenarios where the immune system is compromised (e.g., chemotherapy, HIV, uncontrolled diabetes). Esophageal candidiasis is when these plaques extend into the esophagus, sometimes resulting in dysphagia.

Diagnosis for candidiasis is made by looking in the patient's mouth or esophagus.

Treatment includes prescribed medicated mouthwash or oral medication.

APHTHOUS ULCERS

Aphthous ulcers, also known as canker sores, can be caused by immune abnormalities, nutritional deficiencies, chronic trauma (dentures), allergies, and/or dry mouth. Sometimes aphthous ulcers can be a manifestation of certain inflammatory conditions like inflammatory bowel disease or Behcet's syndrome.

Diagnosis is via observation of the ulcers in the mouth.

Treatment includes addressing the root cause, avoiding dietary triggers and further mechanical trauma, and applying topical analgesics or anesthetics to help relieve pain. More severe, persistent canker sores may require specific medication.

HERPETIC ULCERS

Herpetic ulcers (cold sores) have an additional layer of keratin, unlike aphthous ulcers. Cold sores are mainly caused by herpes simplex virus (HSV) type 1 (although HSV type 2, which is typically associated with genital herpes, can sometimes also cause oral lesions). Most people contract the virus early in life, and after initial infection, the virus remains dormant in the nervous system. These cold sores can reappear from time to time, first appearing as vesicles before rupturing and leaving painful ulcers that take approximately two weeks to heal.

Diagnosis of herpetic ulcers may require specific testing to detect the HSV-1 virus.

Treatment can include antiviral medication, in pill or topical form, which can be prescribed for these cold sores.

ZENKER'S DIVERTICULUM

Zenker's diverticulum is an outpouching (turning inside out) of the esophagus that can occur later in life. In the back of the throat, there is an area of weakness where the wall of the esophagus is not as well supported by muscle, and a pocket can form from the wall of the esophagus. This can cause difficulty with swallowing or bad breath from trapped food.

Diagnosis using a barium swallow X-ray can help identify this condition.

Treatment for these pockets can be via an endoscopic procedure where the wall between the diverticulum and esophagus is divided so the pocket becomes one with the lumen (inside) of the esophagus.

EOSINOPHILIC ESOPHAGITIS

Eosinophilic esophagitis (EoE) describes inflammation of the esophagus lining with eosinophils as the predominant cell type. Eosinophils are one of the main cells of our immune system, commonly associated with allergic conditions. Typically, the esophagus doesn't have many eosinophils present in its lining, but they are present in EoE, triggering an inflammatory response. Symptoms include dysphagia, chest pain, and food impaction requiring procedural removal of food that is stuck in the esophagus, which is often how the condition is initially diagnosed. It is unclear what causes this condition, although food allergies may be involved.

Diagnosis is made via an endoscopy with a biopsy of the esophageal lining to detect an abundance of eosinophils.

Treatment, as for many allergic conditions, is long-standing to maintain remission and may consist of an elimination diet, proton pump inhibitors (PPI; see p179), or topical steroids. Untreated EoE may result in strictures of the esophagus.

ESOPHAGEAL RINGS

Esophageal rings or webs are very common. A mucosal "Schatzki's" ring of the esophagus is likely related to GERD (see p104) and therefore closer to the bottom of the esophagus. Most rings leave an opening wide enough for food to pass through. However, if the diameter of the esophagus is reduced to less than 13mm or so, solid food impactions can occur.

Whereas rings are often acquired, esophageal webs (where only part of the esophagus is obstructed) develop before birth and tend to be in the upper to midesophagus. Sometimes iron deficiency can cause esophageal webs in Plummer-Vinson syndrome, and the webs disappear after the iron deficiency is treated.

Diagnosis can be made using a barium swallow X-ray or by an endoscopy of the upper esophagus.

Treatment for these webs and rings is typically mechanical dilation, acid reduction with PPIs, and at times endoscopic surgery to open the rings up.

ACHALASIA

Achalasia is an esophageal motility disorder, which causes abnormal movement of the esophageal muscles, resulting in dysphagia, chest pain, or heartburn. In achalasia, the lower esophageal sphincter is unable to relax and the esophageal muscles leading up to the sphincter are unable to contract normally (carry out peristalsis) to move food downward.

When the lower esophageal sphincter can relax appropriately but the peristalsis is still impaired, other diagnoses like a distal esophageal spasm or jackhammer esophagus could be present. Jackhammer esophagus is so named because the esophagus contracts so forcefully, and the squeezing is exaggerated and painful.

Diagnosis is made by imaging and an endoscopy to rule out any structural abnormalities in the esophagus first, before undergoing manometry and other motility testing.

Treatment can include medications like smooth muscle relaxants, which may help in the short term but are often ineffective for long-term relief. Although injections of botulinum toxin (Botox) to the lower esophageal sphincter may help with achalasia, the need for repeat procedures also makes this option less appealing. A more reliable treatment procedure for achalasia would be surgical or endoscopic cutting of the sphincter muscle.

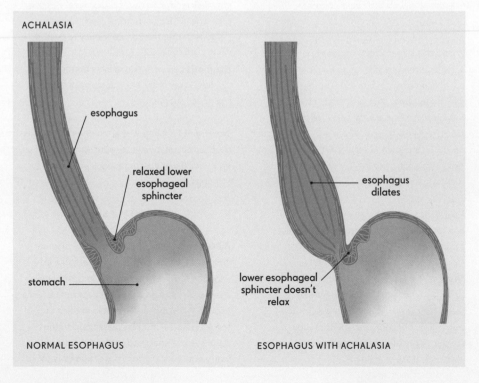

ACHALASIA

esophagus

relaxed lower esophageal sphincter

esophagus dilates

stomach

lower esophageal sphincter doesn't relax

NORMAL ESOPHAGUS

ESOPHAGUS WITH ACHALASIA

ESOPHAGEAL CANCER

Esophageal cancer rates are rising at an alarming rate, having doubled between 2012 and 2019 among those aged 45 to 64. Two main types of esophageal cancer are squamous cell carcinoma (SCC) and adenocarcinoma. Esophageal SCC is found in the upper third or middle of the esophagus and is linked to smoking and alcohol consumption. The most common type of esophageal cancer is adenocarcinoma, found in the lower third of the esophagus often as a result of chronic acid exposure.

Diagnosis For patients with long-standing GERD, screening for Barrett's esophagus, or precancerous changes in the lower portion of the esophagus, is recommended.

Treatment in the past for any precancerous findings would have been an esophagectomy, the surgical removal of part of the esophagus. Today, there are technologies to tackle affected areas in a less invasive way, removing precancerous cells and preventing cancer from developing. While early cancers often do not cause any symptoms, weight loss and dysphagia are common symptoms of esophageal cancer (for both SCC and adenocarcinoma). Once the diagnosis is confirmed via an endoscopy, early small cancers limited to the most superficial layers of the esophageal lining may be removed endoscopically. However, for larger tumors, surgery may be required to remove the affected portion of the esophagus, and chemotherapy and radiotherapy may also be recommended. For tumors that cannot be surgically removed, a metal stent can be installed opening the esophagus to allow food to pass down into the stomach.

DIAPHRAGMATIC HERNIAS

Hernias occur when an organ pushes through a weakness in the muscle or tissue wall. In sliding hiatal and paraesophageal hernias, the stomach protrudes upward through the diaphragm into the chest. The more of the stomach that extends into the chest, the more discomfort and respiratory symptoms a person may experience as there is less room for the lungs to expand.

Diagnosis involves the patient being asked to stand, cough, or strain to check for a bulge. If it is not apparent, then the doctor may request an abdominal ultrasound, CT scan, or MRI.

Treatment for small hiatal hernias is repair endoscopically, whereas for larger hiatal hernias and paraesophageal hernias surgical repair of the opening in the diaphragm is required.

Often the underlying cause for varices is cirrhosis, or scarring of the liver.

MALLORY-WEISS TEARS AND BOERHAAVE SYNDROME

Mallory-Weiss tears happen when the esophagus lining tears and patients can vomit blood (hematemesis). More dramatically in Boerhaave syndrome, the esophageal wall ruptures from forceful vomiting, resulting in severe chest pain.

Diagnosis for Mallory-Weiss tears is made by an upper gastrointestinal endoscopy, whereas a water-soluble contrast swallow test and X-ray is used to diagnose Boerhaave syndrome.

Treatment for both conditions would be urgent surgery to stop the influx of bacteria into the esophagus.

ESOPHAGEAL VARICES

Varices are engorged blood vessels resulting from impaired blood flow through the portal vein, the large blood vessel that carries blood through the liver. Often the underlying cause for varices is cirrhosis, or scarring of the liver. Variceal bleeding is dramatic, with blood squirting from a blood vessel because of the elevated pressure within the vessel.

Diagnosis is made by carrying out an upper gastrointestinal endoscopy.

Treatment in most cases is made endoscopically, treating the bleeding blood vessel with a banding device that deploys rubber bands to constrict the blood vessel.

VARICES
As a varix is at high risk of bleeding, an endoscopist ties off the vessel using a rubber band that stops the blood from leaking.

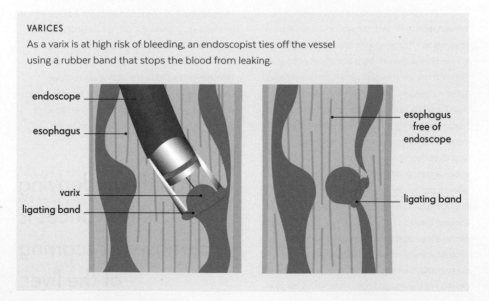

endoscope

esophagus

varix

ligating band

esophagus free of endoscope

ligating band

Stomach

GASTROPARESIS

Gastroparesis is a condition where the stomach empties too slowly. Common causes include diabetes or complications postsurgery, but often the cause is unknown. In patients with long-standing diabetes, the nerves of the stomach are not able to contract properly in response to meals. In patients who have undergone surgery where the vagus nerve is severed, the stomach is also unable to contract or relax to facilitate digestion. Regardless of the cause, patients with gastroparesis usually complain of fullness, abdominal discomfort, nausea, and vomiting.

Diagnosis for gastroparesis is made using an endoscopy to rule out structural causes such as a blockage of stomach outflow. A gastric emptying test is often performed to assess the timing of stomach emptying.

Treatment includes some medications that can help with stomach muscle movement, although some, like metoclopramide, may cause irreversible side effects, such as sudden abnormal movements of the face and body known as tardive dyskinesia, which can develop with long-term use. To help with symptoms, an adjustment in eating habits and anti-nausea medications are commonly recommended. For a more sustainable solution, sometimes gastric stimulators or pacemakers can be implanted. There are also some investigational procedures performed to help muscles relax and allow the stomach to empty more easily.

GASTRIC VOLVULUS

Gastric volvulus occurs when the stomach twists on itself because of lax attachments that usually keep the stomach and its surrounding structures in place. This often happens in conjunction with a diaphragmatic hernia. Gastric volvulus can result in sudden, severe pain in the upper abdomen and retching without bringing up any food. Sudden, acute twisting can lead to compromised blood flow.

Diagnosis may involve imaging tests, such as a CT scan, endoscopy, and a barium swallow to help the radiologist see abnormalities.

Treatment of acute gastric volvulus needs surgical intervention, which involves untwisting the volvulus, fixation of the stomach, and repair of the diaphragmatic hernia.

Gastritis most commonly refers to inflammation of the stomach lining.

HELICOBACTER PYLORI (H. PYLORI) INFECTION

Helicobacter pylori (*H. pylori*) **infection** is described as the most common bacterial infection in the world, with estimates of at least 50 percent of the world's population being infected with the bacteria. Diseases linked to *H. pylori* infection include gastritis, peptic ulcer disease, gastric cancer, and gastric lymphoma. The identification of this bacteria has fundamentally changed the thinking of how bacteria could be linked to cancer and has transformed how gastric ulcers are treated since surgical resection was sometimes performed just to cure an ulcer in the past. Exactly how the bacteria is transmitted is unclear but human-to-human transmission through gastric or fecal contents seems likely.

Diagnosis involves testing for the bacteria and may include stool tests, blood tests, breath tests, or an endoscopy with a biopsy of the gastric mucosa.

Treatment typically involves a short course of antibiotics and a PPI.

GASTRITIS

Gastritis most commonly refers to inflammation of the stomach lining. Most cases are chronic, with *H. pylori* infection the most common cause. There are many other causes of chronic gastritis, including inflammatory conditions and other bacteria and viruses. Often patients with chronic gastritis have no symptoms, although these may develop with more severe inflammation that can lead to stomach ulcers.

Diagnosis is often made following an endoscopy and a biopsy of the stomach lining.

Treatment includes antibiotics and antacids and dietary changes to ease the symptoms.

In chronic atrophic gastritis, the body cannot keep up with cell turnover from chronic inflammation and the mucosa thins. Although this can be caused by chronic infection, it can also be caused by an autoimmune condition where the body develops antibodies against parietal cells and intrinsic factor. Parietal cells secrete gastric acid and a substance called intrinsic factor, which helps transport and absorb vitamin B12. When parietal cells are destroyed, acid production is halted. These changes then lead to nutritional deficiencies and precancerous changes.

PEPTIC ULCERS

Peptic ulcers are found in the stomach and duodenum. (Gastric ulcers are specific to the stomach). Ulcers are formed when inflammation breaks down the stomach lining. The most common causes are a *H. pylori* bacterial infection and the use of nonsteroidal anti-inflammatory drugs (NSAID). Smoking, stress, and alcohol use are seen as potential risk factors, too. It is thought that the defense mechanism of the stomach lining is suppressed by all. The most common complication of ulcers is bleeding.

Diagnosis of gastric ulcers can be made in several ways and includes testing blood, breath, and stool, then via an endoscopy.

Treatment includes medication to suppress acid production and endoscopic intervention when the ulcer is also sampled to assess for *H. pylori* infection and cancerous changes. Depending on the nature of the bleeding, a variety of treatment methods are used, including clips, cautery, or injection of vasoconstricting medication to stop the bleeding.

Treatment for gastric cancer detected early (when the cancer may be limited to the most superficial layers of the stomach lining) can include an endoscopic technique called endoscopic submucosal dissection, to remove cancerous tissue. However, surgery may be required in many cases, along with chemotherapy and radiotherapy.

GASTRIC CANCER

Gastric cancer remains a top cause of cancer death in the world, with an estimated 800,000 cancer deaths a year, the majority occurring in Asia. There are two types of gastric cancer: intestinal and diffuse. The intestinal type is more common and thought to be associated with environmental and dietary factors and occurs in older individuals, versus the diffuse type, which affects younger people. Known risk factors for gastric adenocarcinoma include *H. pylori* infection, chronic atrophic gastritis, cigarette smoking, and certain genetic conditions. The greater prevalence of gastric cancer in Asia has been attributed to higher rates of *H. pylori* infection and greater consumption of foods high in salt and nitrates, although this dietary link is not conclusive.

Diagnosis is often made late with a third of cases metastatic at the time of diagnosis as symptoms of gastric cancer are common to other digestive conditions.

Gastric cancer remains a top cause of deaths in the world, with an estimated 800,000 cancer deaths per year.

Intestines

IRRITABLE BOWEL SYNDROME (IBS)

Irritable bowel syndrome (IBS) is a chronic condition where patients suffer from altered bowel movements, frequency, stool consistency, and abdominal pain. The prevalence of IBS is between 7 to 16 percent in the US. For as common as it is, very little is still known about IBS and the cause remains unclear. Some studies suggest it is a disorder of the gut-brain interaction, with abnormal sensitivity of the gut, and abnormal responses to signals received. The most recent definition of IBS defines it as recurrent abdominal pain for at least one day per week over a three-month period with a change in bowel movements and stool appearance. Depending on the predominant symptom, IBS can be further divided into constipation-predominant IBS (IBS-C), diarrhea-predominant IBS (IBS-D), mixed IBS (IBS-M) or IBS unclassified (IBS-U), where IBS is diagnosed but symptoms fall outside of the other categories.

Diagnosis for IBS is made by assessing whether you meet the diagnostic criteria as outlined in the illustration below. Unfortunately, apart from meeting certain diagnostic criteria, there is no specific lab or imaging test that can tell us whether someone has IBS. The main purpose of any testing of that sort is to make sure there's no other diagnosis or explanation for an individual's symptoms.

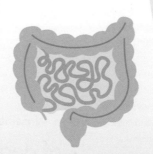

SUBTYPES OF IBS

IBS-C (CONSTIPATION PREDOMINANT)

constipation is the main symptom, alongside:

abdominal discomfort and/or pain

bloating

straining to have a bowel movement

IBS-D (DIARRHEA PREDOMINANT)

diarrhea is the main symptom, along with:

abdominal pain and/or discomfort

sudden urges to go to the bathroom

gas

IBS-M (MIXED)

symptoms of both IBS-C and IBS-D

IBS-U (UNCLASSIFIED)

symptoms fall outside of the other IBS categories

Treatment for IBS varies depending on what the predominant symptom is. For bloating, one of the main approaches is a low-FODMAP diet (see p25). Trained dietary professionals can help figure out which of the FODMAPs may be triggering IBS symptoms. Peppermint tea and medications to limit intestinal spasms may also help in relieving these symptoms. Treatment geared toward symptoms of constipation (see pp112-113) or diarrhea may be recommended (see pp114-115).

SMALL INTESTINAL BACTERIAL OVERGROWTH (SIBO)

Small intestinal bacterial overgrowth (SIBO) is an overgrowth of bacteria in the intestine. These bacteria can have various effects, including injuring the intestinal mucosa through loss of brush border enzymes, competing for nutrients in the gut, and further fermenting carbohydrates and producing by-products that interfere with normal gut metabolism and cause symptoms as a result. The exact cause of SIBO is unclear, but there may be multiple contributors like changes in the stomach acid environment that usually eradicates certain bacteria, changes in the intestinal motility that allows bacteria to proliferate, altered intestinal anatomy after surgery, or loss of other protective mechanisms.

Diagnosis of SIBO is made indirectly, using breath tests that measure elevated levels of hydrogen or methane. These tests are not always accurate.

Treatment for suspected SIBO may include antibiotics to eradicate excess bacteria.

FOOD POISONING

Food poisoning is an illness caused by eating food contaminated by bacteria, bacterial toxins, viruses, parasites, or chemicals found in edible substances. Medications (those reducing stomach acid) or underlying conditions (like liver disease or immune deficiencies) may predispose some people to food poisoning. Often symptoms include abdominal pain, diarrhea, nausea, and/or vomiting. Common bacteria associated with food poisoning include *Salmonella, Campylobacter, Clostridium. perfringens, Shigella,* and *E. coli.* Mass production of foods can lead to outbreaks of food poisoning, and antibiotic use in the meat industry has led to bacteria becoming increasingly resistant to treatment.

Diagnosis is made based on symptoms present, which, depending on the bacteria present, can begin anywhere between 1 to 48 hours after eating contaminated food.

Treatment aims to replace the fluids lost with vomiting or diarrhea, as dehydration is a common concern. After infecting the bloodstream, some bacteria may go on to infect heart valves or even the brain. Botulism is another (relatively rare) example where life-threatening muscle paralysis might result, possibly requiring mechanical ventilation to help patients breathe.

CELIAC DISEASE

Celiac disease is an autoimmune condition where the body develops antibodies against gluten. These antibodies then attack the intestinal mucosa, causing it to flatten and lose its absorptive fingerlike projections (or villi). Some grains contain gluten (like wheat, rye, and barley), while others do not (like corn, rice, and millet). Celiac disease can affect virtually all organs. Some patients present with gastrointestinal (GI) symptoms, including diarrhea, steatorrhea (greasy stools), bloating, and flatulence. Other more subtle effects include weight loss, vague abdominal discomfort, anemia, osteopenia, and neurological symptoms. Other conditions are associated with celiac disease, including an itchy skin rash called dermatitis herpetiformis and other autoimmune diseases.

Diagnosis of celiac disease involves an intestinal biopsy, where the loss of intestinal villi can be seen. Celiac-related antibody blood tests are used for both diagnosis and monitoring of the disease.

WORN-DOWN INTESTINES

In celiac disease, exposure to gluten causes autoantibodies to abnormally develop triggering an inflammatory response that results in villous atrophy, or flattening of the absorptive lining of the intestine. By avoiding gluten, normal villi will be restored.

NORMAL INTESTINAL VILLI

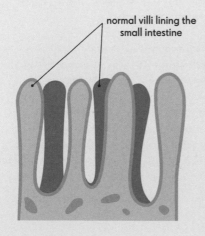

normal villi lining the small intestine

CELIAC DISEASE

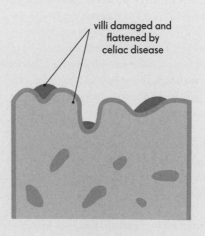

villi damaged and flattened by celiac disease

Treatment involves a lifelong commitment to a gluten-free diet, which can be challenging, especially as many processed foods contain hidden gluten, which could prevent the disease from improving. Additional treatment may be required in those with refractory disease, and T-cell lymphoma should be ruled out given the increased risk of this malignancy with celiac disease.

INTESTINAL HERNIAS

Intestinal hernias occur when loops of the intestine protrude through weak areas of a muscular wall.

Diagnosis is via examination; hernias can be visible depending on their location. Inguinal hernias occur in the groin, whereas umbilical hernias protrude through the belly button.

Treatment for benign hernias can be weight loss and avoiding exertion like heavy lifting or abdominal strain during a bowel movement. If complications of hernia occur, such as the intestine becoming trapped in the opening (incarcerated hernia), which can potentially compromise blood flow (strangulated hernia) emergency surgical intervention may be required.

CROHN'S DISEASE (CD)

Crohn's disease (CD) is one of the two major forms of inflammatory bowel disease and can affect any part of the gut from mouth to anus. It is a chronic condition with "skip lesions," meaning the gut is affected in a discontinuous fashion. Patients often present with abdominal pain, loose stools, anemia, weight loss, and even fever.

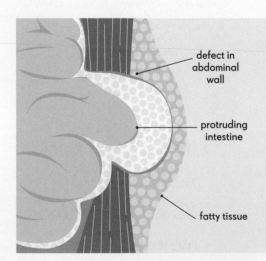

defect in abdominal wall

protruding intestine

fatty tissue

PROTRUDING LINING
Defects in the abdominal wall allow loops of intestine to poke through and often slide back and forth. However, if the intestine becomes trapped, surgery may be necessary to move them back into place and repair the abdominal wall, especially if intestinal blood flow is compromised (strangulation).

Diagnosis can be reached with endoscopy, histopathology (biopsy findings under a microscope), and cross-sectional imaging. Because the disease affects all layers of the gut wall, the disease can result in ulcerations or full-thickness complications like fistulas (connections that form between two hollow structures, such as the vagina and bladder, or two loops of intestine). Scarring may also occur, leading to strictures of the intestine. Some patients develop perianal symptoms, including skin tags, fistulas, and abscesses. There are also other symptoms that can originate from outside the intestine, including joint pains, skin lesions (pyoderma gangrenosum, erythema nodosum), and even clinical findings in the eyes (like episcleritis or uveitis).

Treatment aims to drive the disease into remission, and treatment varies by acuity, severity, and location of the disease.

There is no cure for Crohn's disease, and the cause is not well understood but is thought to involve genes, bacteria, and environmental factors. Acute flares of the disease sometimes require corticosteroids to control the flare. Other medications include anti-inflammatory aminosalicylates, immunomodulators like azathioprine or 6-mercaptopurine, and antibody biologic therapies such as infliximab, adalimumab, vedolizumab, and others are often used for long-term treatment. Surgery may be required for fistulas, abscesses, strictures, and other complications of Crohn's disease.

ULCERATIVE COLITIS (UC)

Ulcerative colitis (UC) is the other of the two main forms of inflammatory bowel disease. Unlike Crohn's disease (CD), UC affects only the full length of the colon or just the distal part.

Diagnosis, as for CD, involves a combination of endoscopy, imaging, and histopathology, which would demonstrate inflammation that is typically limited to the mucosal layer. Patients can present with diarrhea, rectal bleeding, abdominal pain, and urgency to pass a stool. Similar to CD, there can be manifestations of the disease outside the intestine, including joint disease, skin symptoms, and eye disease. Onset is often slow and gradual, although it can sometimes be severe and require colectomy (removal of the colon) on initial presentation and is characterized by intermittent flares.

Treatment varies according to the severity of the disease. As with CD, the goal of medical therapy for UC is to induce and maintain remission. Medication choice is driven by the acuity, severity, and extent of the disease.

Like CD, the goal of medical therapy for UC is to induce and maintain remission.

Corticosteroids are used as first-line therapy in moderate to severe flares but are not intended for chronic use. Aminosalicylates, immunomodulators, and biological therapies are also used.

Approximately 30 percent of patients require a colectomy after 25 years with UC. For those who require surgery, often it is a partial or complete resection of the colon. While the small intestine and the remaining colon can sometimes be reconnected, at times they remain disconnected. The upstream small bowel is often redirected toward the skin (ileostomy), allowing passage of waste externally, while any remaining colon is fashioned into a pouch. This pouch can also become diseased, at times from recurrent UC or other possible consequences of surgery.

DIVERTICULAR DISEASE

Diverticular disease is when pockets (diverticula) develop in the intestinal lining, and protrude past the muscle layer of the gut. The cause of diverticula remains unclear but could be due to intestinal wall weakness with age, increased pressure within the intestine, or changes in intestinal motility. Symptoms may develop when these pockets become inflamed or infected (diverticulitis).

Diagnosis can involve giving blood and poop samples and tests such as a colonoscopy or a CT scan.

Treatment of mild cases can involve managing symptoms with oral antibiotics in an outpatient setting, although more severe cases may require inpatient hospitalization with intravenous antibiotics. A colonoscopy is often recommended after diverticulitis to make sure the underlying trigger for the diverticulitis isn't an undiagnosed colorectal cancer. Diverticular

COLONIC DIVERTICULA
Potholes along a highway is a good analogy for colonic diverticula . Diverticulosis describes the presence of these diverticula, but diverticulitis is when one of these potholes becomes inflamed. Serious cases may require surgery to remove the segment of colon, especially if inflammation over time leads to narrowing (strictures).

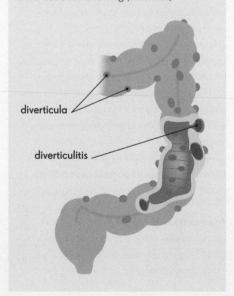

diverticula

diverticulitis

bleeding is a common cause of significant lower GI bleeding. It's unclear what causes these pockets to bleed, and most diverticular bleeds stop on their own. In stable patients, a colonoscopy may be performed to examine for other causes of bleeding or to stop the bleed. In unstable patients, management with embolization (block a vessel with plugging material) by interventional radiology specialists or surgery for colonic resection may be required.

APPENDICITIS

Appendicitis is the most common acute abdominal emergency in developed countries, with more than 250,000 appendectomies performed each year in the US. The cause of an inflamed appendix remains unknown; among leading theories is the blockage of the appendix with a stool ball or some other growth or infection of the appendix.

Typically, patients present with right lower quadrant pain, which can be accompanied by nausea, vomiting, and potentially fever and chills, especially if the appendix is perforated. A perforated appendix can result in more serious complications, including peritonitis or abscess.

Diagnosis of appendicitis is confirmed with blood tests and imaging.

Treatment is an appendectomy (surgical removal of the appendix), most of which is performed using a laparoscopic approach (through small incisions in the abdomen).

HEMORRHOIDS (PILES)

Hemorrhoids (piles) are enlarged blood vessels between the anal mucosa and the muscular sphincter. Located above the dentate line that divides the upper and lower parts of the anal canal, internal hemorrhoids are not usually painful unless they clot. They are thought to result from constipation and increased time spent sitting on the toilet. Piles can also bleed, swell, and prolapse outside the body.

Diagnosis can be confirmed with a physical examination.

Treatment typically initially consists of changes to dietary habits and fluid intake to promote smooth passage of bowel movements and minimize time straining or sitting on the toilet. For larger internal hemorrhoids, patients may be offered a surgical procedure to remove them. External hemorrhoids occur at the anal verge and can be painful, especially with thrombosis. Over-the-counter topical creams can provide temporary relief by shrinking down the enlarged blood vessels, and submerging these hemorrhoids in sitz baths may provide symptomatic relief. Pain usually subsides after several days, but prolonged painful hemorrhoids may require a procedure to remove any clots.

COLON OR COLORECTAL CANCER

Colon or colorectal cancer is cancer of the large intestine, which includes both the colon and the rectum. Worldwide, it is the third most diagnosed cancer with an estimated 2 million people diagnosed in 2020 alone. In the US, it is the third leading cause of cancer deaths among both men and women. Fortunately, colon cancer is one of the few cancers that can often be prevented through early detection by regular screening.

Diagnosis can be made through screening. The rate of colorectal cancer diagnoses has risen among individuals younger than 50 years old in recent decades. As a result, recommendations for screening for average-risk individuals in the US were recently revised to begin at age 45. Despite celebrities promoting screening, rates are less than ideal. While colonoscopy remains the gold standard (for the ability to see, locate, and remove potential precancerous growths on the spot), there are also other screening options for those who cannot tolerate a colonoscopy. Many patients with colorectal cancer often lack obvious symptoms. Others may note a sudden change in regularity or consistency of bowel movement or fatigue resulting from anemia (low blood counts) from slow blood loss. Blood in the stool or changes in stool color also requires further investigation. Like many other cancers, unintended weight loss is a red flag that triggers doctors to look for potential cancer.

While the concept may seem simple, performing a colonoscopy is not an easy task—for both the patient and the surgeon. Patients have to "prep" their colon by drinking a bowel preparation designed to fully flush out the colon. Some find this an uncomfortable procedure. However, it is particularly important because, without clean surfaces within the colon, it is difficult for the surgeon to see what lies under any food residue or stool.

For the surgeon performing the colonoscopy, maneuvering a long floppy scope safely through a windy colon takes dexterity and years of practice. Looking carefully behind folds, identifying subtle cancers, and differentiating them from harmless findings can be tough. Precancerous polyps can range from tiny bumps to large tumors that can completely obstruct the colon.

The purpose of a colonoscopy is to identify and remove precancerous growths called polyps before they become cancers. Polyps like tubular adenomas, villous adenomas, and sessile serrated polyps are all considered precancerous,

Colon cancer is one of the few cancers that can often be prevented through early detection by regular screening.

but the risk of them turning into cancer depends on the size and the degree of precancerous changes. Other polyps like hyperplastic polyps and inflammatory polyps in the colon do not always carry the potential for developing into cancer. During a colonoscopy, the surgeon will assess the various features of the polyp to determine how to best address it.

Treatment of colon cancer aims to remove the growths. Typically, small lumps and bumps that appear, such as a precancerous polyp, are removed by plucking them off using forceps or by throwing a snare (a lassolike tool) over the polyp and cutting it off. More advanced techniques in recent years have facilitated the safe removal of bigger polyps that historically would have required surgical removal of entire sections of the colon. One of the most rapidly growing areas within gastroenterology today is a technique called endoscopic submucosal dissection (ESD), where doctors lift the large polyp off its deeper layers and carve it out. Even early-stage cancers, limited to the inner layer of the colon wall, can be removed in this fashion avoiding invasive surgery.

Innovation around colonoscopy is still happening! Artificial intelligence is becoming increasingly available to help doctors identify polyps during colonoscopy, reducing the chance of missed polyps.

ANAL CANCER

Anal cancer is relatively rare among GI cancers, and most are squamous cell cancers, though other types like adenocarcinoma and melanoma can also occur. Many of these anal cancers are thought to be related to human papilloma virus (HPV) infection.

Diagnosis can be made by screening, with tests such as a physical examination, blood test, or biopsy.

Treatment can include chemotherapy, radiotherapy, and surgical removal of the cancer.

• COLON POLYP SYNDROMES •

In familial adenomatous polyposis (FAP) syndrome, patients are prone to developing polyps due to a baseline mutation of the APC gene. When left untreated, FAP carries a 100% progression to colorectal cancer. Other variants of FAP may include manifestations outside the intestine including tumors in the bone, thyroid, adrenal glands, brain, and other organs. Early monitoring with upper endoscopy, colonoscopy, and other imaging studies are recommended to screen for cancer. Lynch syndrome is a condition where the DNA repair mechanism that normally serves to correct mistakes in DNA can lead to a higher risk of colon cancer. Regular screening colonoscopies are also recommended, starting at an earlier age.

ANAL FISSURES

Anal fissures are tears in the lining of the anus, often presenting with intense sharp pain and bleeding. While fissures can occur after the passage of a large, firm bowel movement, it is possible the anus itself may be predisposed to injury from hypertonic sphincter activity (abnormally high muscle tone causing constant contraction) causing poor blood flow, leading to pain.

Diagnosis is made by discussing your symptoms with your doctor and getting a physical examination if necessary.

Treatment may initially begin with dietary modifications to promote softer bowel movements, but interventions may also include topical medications to relax the sphincter muscle or botulinum toxin injection into the area. Surgery may be performed to cut the sphincter if the fissure remains chronic.

PROTEIN-LOSING ENTEROPATHY

Multiple disorders cause protein-rich fluid to leak into the gut through mucosal ulcerations (as seen in Crohn's disease), loss of protein through cell shedding or vascular changes (as with Lupus), or through leakage of protein-rich lymph associated with blockage of the lymphatic system. Low levels of specific proteins like albumin and immunoglobulins (antibodies) are often detected in the blood and can manifest as edema (swelling).

Diagnosis of protein-losing enteropathy can be made by measuring stool levels of specific proteins like alpha-1-antitrypsin protein before looking for an underlying cause with endoscopy or other imaging studies.

Treatment aims to resolve the underlying cause of the disorder.

MALABSORPTION

Lactose malabsorption (often known as lactose intolerance) occurs when there is a deficiency in the lactase enzyme in the intestinal lining that causes diarrhea, abdominal cramping, and bloating. Symptoms may vary in severity depending on how much of the enzyme is lost, other concomitant conditions, and the amount of lactose that is consumed.

Fat malabsorption can occur with pancreatic insufficiency and the lack of enzymes to process consumed fat.

• SHORT BOWEL SYNDROME (SBS) •

At least 39 in (100 cm) of the jejunum is typically required for micronutrient absorption and fluid and electrolyte balance. Patients who've had long segments of their intestines affected by disease or removed surgically may suffer from short bowel syndrome as there is insufficient surface area to absorb fluid and nutrients.

Bile acid malabsorption may also lead to fat malabsorption in certain conditions where segments of the intestine have been surgically removed.

Diagnosis of malabsorption can be sought via blood, stool, or breath tests or a biopsy of the small intestine lining.

Treatment aims to replace the nutrients and fluids lost by malabsorption and address the root cause with medication and changes to diet.

Lactose intolerance occurs when there is a deficiency in the lactase enzyme in the intestinal lining.

ILEUS

Ileus is a condition where the intestine fails to push food forward, leading to a functional blockage of the intestines. Causes include anesthesia, effects after surgery, opiate medications, electrolyte abnormalities, inflammation, and more. Patients with ileus present with abdominal pain, belly distention, nausea, and vomiting.

Diagnosis can be made via imaging, which may reveal dilated loops of bowel without evidence of a true mechanical blockage.

Treatment may involve decompressing the bowel by suctioning out gut contents through a nasogastric tube, bowel rest, and intravenous fluids. Over time, addressing the underlying cause of allowing time for recovery will allow intestinal function to resume.

OGILVIE'S SYNDROME

Ogilvie's syndrome causes dilation of the colon as a result of a sudden loss of function of the colon in the absence of a blockage. Causes include trauma, infections, and cardiac causes like myocardial infarction or heart failure.

Diagnosis can be made with imaging to see if the colon is significantly dilated and at risk of bursting.

Treatment for Ogilvie's syndrome may include medications like neostigmine to restore colonic movement. As a last resort, surgery may be required to resect part of the colon to relieve pressure, although this can be risky and is associated with higher rates of poor outcomes.

INTESTINAL PROTOZOA

Protozoa infections occur through fecal-oral transmission, and while most patients don't have symptoms, about 10 to 20 percent of individuals may develop invasive disease where the organism invades the colonic lining through the bloodstream to go on and invade other organs. *Giardia intestinalis* is the most identified parasite in the US and can be transmitted through food, water, or person to person. Infection can range from asymptomatic to causing chronic diarrhea, fatigue, abdominal cramping, and flatulence.

Diagnosis is best sought through colonoscopy, with biopsy of the colonic mucosa, which would reveal the organism.

Treatment is with antiparasitic medications.

INTESTINAL WORMS

There are three general categories of worms: roundworms (nematodes), tapeworms (cestodes), and trematodes (flukes or flatworms). Roundworms enter the body through contaminated food or the skin, passing through the intestinal wall into the bloodstream. Large numbers of worms can lead to an intestinal obstruction or travel elsewhere in the body, causing further problems. Among tapeworms, the largest parasite to infect humans is the *Diphyllobothrium* species, which can be 40 ft (12 m) long. Intestinal, liver, and blood flukes can also cause infection, chronic inflammation, or even cancer depending on which organ they affect.

Diagnosis can be made from testing stool or blood samples.

Treatment can often be as simple as a single dose of medication.

INTESTINAL WORMS AND PROTOZOA

roundworm

protozoa

fluke

tapeworm

INFECTIOUS DIARRHEA

Infectious diarrhea and dysentery (bloody diarrhea) can be caused by bacteria like *Shigella*, *Yersinia*, or *E. coli*, as well as certain parasites. Depending on the cause, stool quality and frequency may vary. Dehydration may also occur due to significant fluid loss.

Diagnosis can be made with a stool sample.

Treatment aims to replenish lost water and electrolytes.

Liver

CIRRHOSIS

Cirrhosis is the final process of liver injury from many causes, where normal liver tissue is replaced by scar tissue. The most common causes of cirrhosis in the US are fatty liver disease, chronic alcohol use, and hepatitis C infection. Cirrhosis is the eighth most common cause of death in the US, and median life expectancy is around 9 to 12 years for those with compensated cirrhosis (or without major complications).

Diagnosis of cirrhosis by examining liver tissue from a biopsy is considered the gold standard. But there are often many physical findings, too, that suggest underlying cirrhosis, and when blood tests and imaging are available, a biopsy is not always required for diagnosis. There are also noninvasive ultrasound-based imaging tests that measure the stiffness of the liver.

Treatment for those with "compensated" cirrhosis includes regular screening for liver cancer (hepatocellular carcinoma) and surveillance of esophageal varices. Vaccinations against other preventable hepatitis viruses are also recommended to prevent secondary injury.

DISEASE THAT TYPICALLY LEAD TO LIVER CIRRHOSIS

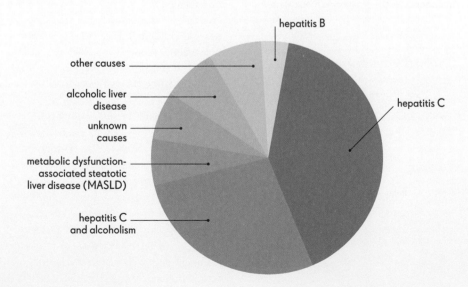

hepatitis B

other causes

alcoholic liver disease

unknown causes

metabolic dysfunction-associated steatotic liver disease (MASLD)

hepatitis C and alcoholism

hepatitis C

Many of the complications that arise from cirrhosis that require attention are results of portal hypertension. The only definitive treatment for cirrhosis is a liver transplant. Like many other organ transplant evaluation protocols, there is a rigorous process evaluating candidacy for transplantation considering prognosis, and social support, among other criteria.

METABOLIC DYSFUNCTION-ASSOCIATED STEATOTIC LIVER DISEASE (MASLD)

Metabolic dysfunction-associated steatotic liver disease (MASLD) refers to fatty deposits in liver cells, a condition closely associated with obesity, diabetes, and other metabolic disorders. Cases of MASLD are increasing, affecting a quarter of the world's population. The disease can become progressively severe, causing liver inflammation (nonalcoholic steatohepatitis or "NASH") and later fibrosis (scarring) that can lead to cirrhosis and possibly cancer.

Diagnosis of MASLD can be difficult as there are often no symptoms until later in the disease. The gold standard of diagnosing fatty liver disease is a liver biopsy, but fatty liver and its consequences can be detected on other forms of imaging.

Treatment is mainly centered around weight loss and treatment of associated metabolic conditions.

VIRAL HEPATITIS

Viral hepatitis can be caused by various viruses or liver inflammation. These viruses include commonly known hepatitis viruses A, B, C, D, and E but also other viruses like Epstein–Barr virus (EBV), Cytomegalovirus (CMV), and herpes simplex virus (HSV). These viruses can cause inflammation of the liver, and although infection can be cleared quickly, as in the case of hepatitis A, hepatitis B or C can cause a chronic infection and persistent inflammation leading to scarring that eventually may progress to cirrhosis and possibly liver cancer.

Depending on the virus, there are various ways to prevent infection. Hepatitis A or E are usually transmitted through contaminated food or water, so simply handwashing could prevent infection. For hepatitis B and C, where transmission is often through blood or semen, sharing needles or unprotected sexual contact are risk factors. Hepatitis D occurs only together with hepatitis B, so the same strategies for avoiding hepatitis B would apply to hepatitis D.

• DRUG-INDUCED HEPATITIS •

While high doses of acetaminophen (paracetamol) is a common cause of drug-induced hepatitis, there are a wide variety of other medications that can lead, on rare occasions, to drug-induced hepatitis. Certain herbs, such as kava and skullcap, can also cause liver inflammation.

Diagnosis of the type of viral hepatitis can be confirmed with blood tests, as can the severity of the infection and whether it is active or dormant.

Treatment for chronic viral hepatitis, especially for hepatitis C, has improved in recent years. Previously, interferon-based treatments were poorly tolerated with limited effectiveness. But the introduction of direct-acting antivirals in the early 2010s resulted in an eradication rate approaching 100 percent in hepatitis C cases. For hepatitis B, there is technically no cure, but there are antiviral treatments to keep it at bay. For patients who require immunosuppressive therapy like chemotherapy, it is important that patients are screened for hepatitis B infection to prevent it from flaring when the immune system is compromised. There is not specific treatment for hepatitis A, except to rest and stay hydrated, and avoiding substances that stress the liver, such as alcohol and smoking. Typically, no treatment is needed for hepatitis E, unless there is a history of a weakened immune system.

AUTOIMMUNE HEPATITIS

Autoimmune hepatitis is a long-term liver disease, which occurs when the body's immune response develops autoantibodies that attacks the liver, leading to chronic inflammation. There are two types: type 1 and type 2, characterized by two different autoantibodies. The disease can progress to liver fibrosis and cirrhosis over time. Depending on the severity of the condition, symptoms of autoimmune liver disease can include fatigue and jaundice, and other symptoms associated with cirrhosis.

Diagnosis is made from blood tests that detect autoantibodies, and a liver biopsy may also show specific inflammatory patterns.

Treatment typically consists of steroids and other immunosuppressants to reduce the inflammatory response.

LIVER TUMORS

Liver tumors can be either benign (noncancerous) or malignant (cancerous). The most common malignant tumors are hepatocellular carcinoma (HCC), which can be associated with underlying liver diseases such as cirrhosis as well as chronic viral hepatitis due to hepatitis B or C. Like other cancers, without treatment, the tumors can metastasize (spread).

Diagnosis for HCC can be via a biopsy; diagnoses can often be made with imaging and clinical features alone. An elevated level of the serum tumor marker alpha fetoprotein (AFP) is sometimes found via blood tests and can support a diagnosis.

Treatment options include surgical resection, liver transplantation, ablation (removal), chemoembolization (to deliver medication and block off the vessels that feed the tumor), or chemotherapy and other molecular therapies.

PORTAL HYPERTENSION

Portal hypertension is elevated pressure in the portal vein, the main blood vessel returning blood from the intestines back to the heart. It is a common complication of cirrhosis. The elevated pressure manifests in several different ways, many of which are seen with advanced cirrhosis where blood circulation is impacted by disease. These signs are not unique to cirrhosis; increased pressure may also be due to local tumors or circulatory problems further "downstream" like heart failure. With increased portal pressure, blood vessels in the esophagus can become engorged, causing esophageal varices. Variceal bleeding can be dramatic and is an emergency as blood loss can be rapid due to high portal pressure. Another consequence of is ascites, which is fluid trapped in the abdomen.

Diagnosis is made via blood tests, and by imaging tests that show blood flow.

Treatment includes medications to help patients urinate extra fluid to alleviate discomfort, but a paracentesis (where a needle is inserted through the skin to drain the fluid) can also be performed. This fluid is at increased risk of getting infected, a condition called spontaneous bacterial peritonitis, which requires antibiotic therapy. As fluid seeps out of the blood circulation into areas where fluid doesn't belong, some parts of the body assume the body is in a chronically dehydrated state and attempt to rectify the situation, causing dysfunctional changes in blood circulation that can progress to kidney failure, a serious condition called hepatorenal syndrome. When cirrhosis affects blood circulation through the liver, the body shunts the blood away into other vessels that bypass the liver. This allows certain neurotoxins (namely ammonia) that normally get filtered out to travel to the brain, leading to a condition called portosystemic encephalopathy (sometimes known as hepatic encephalopathy).

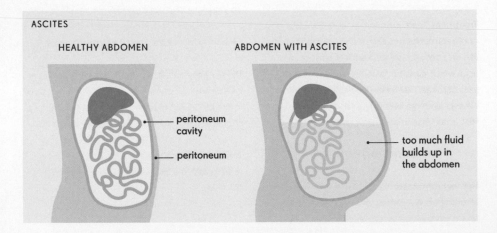

ASCITES

HEALTHY ABDOMEN   ABDOMEN WITH ASCITES

peritoneum cavity

peritoneum

too much fluid builds up in the abdomen

While ammonia production is a normal part of metabolism, when it reaches the brain, it can lead to disorientation, agitation, disrupted sleep, and somnolence. If uncontrolled, it can also lead to coma. Patients are often treated with lactulose to promote bowel movements to clear these toxins, or rifaximin (a nonabsorbable antibiotic).

PRIMARY BILIARY CHOLANGITIS (PBC)

Primary biliary cholangitis is a chronic autoimmune liver disease that affects the bile ducts in the liver, leading to inflammation and impaired flow of bile and eventual destruction of the ducts. Early in the disease, symptoms may be vague, including fatigue or itchiness of the skin, but over time jaundice, abdominal pain, and malabsorption of fat-soluble vitamins may develop.

Diagnosis can be made by detecting anti-mitochondrial antibodies (AMA) in the blood.

Treatment There is no known cure for PBC, and treatment typically consists of medications like urosdeoxycholic acid and/or obeticholic acid, which aims to delay the progression of liver damage. Ultimately some patients may have to undergo liver transplantation, though PBC may recur in the transplanted liver.

HEMOCHROMATOSIS

Hemochromatosis is an inherited disease resulting from a genetic mutation that causes an excess buildup of iron levels in the body leading to iron deposits in various organs. Symptoms include fatigue, joint pain, or in severe cases enlargement of the liver or heart. Secondary hemochromatosis is the result of excessive iron in the diet or from having multiple blood tranfusions to treat an underlying condition, such as sickle cell disease.

Diagnosis of both primary and secondary hemochromatosis is made from taking blood tests and possibly another test to check whether your DNA carries the gene involved.

Treatment is phlebotomy to remove excess iron, which needs to be done regularly, or medication (chelation therapy) to reduce the level of iron.

WILSON DISEASE

Wilson disease is caused by a gene mutation, which leads to excess copper in the liver and brain, among other organs. Copper deposits in the liver can lead to cirrhosis, and in the brain and nervous system, deposits can result in tremors, dystonia, dysphagia, and other neurological and psychiatric manifestations.

Diagnosis can be made by measuring a protein called ceruloplasmin that usually binds to copper in the blood, or by doing an eye test to look for a characteristic copper deposit in the cornea.

Treatment typically starts with a medication to help with the excretion of copper from the body.

Pancreas

ACUTE PANCREATITIS

Acute pancreatitis or acute inflammation of the pancreas is one of the most common GI causes of hospital admission in the US. Gallstones and alcohol use are the two most common causes, with medications, trauma, high triglyceride levels, and hereditary conditions being less common. The pancreas is a sensitive organ, and even endoscopic retrograde cholangiopancreatography (ERC) procedures intended to remove gallstones in the bile duct can irritate the neighboring pancreas.

Whether it's a blockage by a gallstone of the drainage of pancreatic juices into the intestine or direct injury to the pancreas, such as alcohol abuse, a cascade of events is triggered leading to the activation of digestive enzymes that are normally meant to digest food in the intestine. These digestive enzymes can wreak havoc and destroy not only the pancreas itself but also surrounding blood vessels and other structures. Most cases tend to be mild and resolve within days; however, some severe cases of pancreatitis can be life-threatening, especially when a systemic inflammatory response causes other organs to fail.

The main symptom of pancreatitis is upper abdominal pain, often radiating to the back and sometimes relieved by leaning forward, as well as nausea and vomiting.

Diagnosis is made from a combination of blood tests (namely serum lipase) and imaging demonstrating an inflamed pancreas.

Treatment is mainly focused on replenishing fluid losses, preventing the worsening of the condition, and managing complications (like draining infected fluid collections). If gallstones are deemed to be the cause, urgent gallbladder removal is recommended.

CHRONIC PANCREATITIS

Chronic pancreatitis or chronic inflammation of the pancreas eventually leads to irreversible destruction of the pancreas. While long-standing alcohol use is a common cause of chronic pancreatitis, only a small fraction of people who drink alcohol regularly develop the condition. Smoking and other autoimmune and genetic conditions (like cystic fibrosis) may also increase the risk of chronic pancreatitis. It's not fully understood why or how chronic pancreatitis develops, but one explanation is that ongoing injury to the pancreas leads to premature activation of the digestive enzymes resulting in cell death that is ultimately replaced by scar tissue (fibrosis). As more of the pancreas is damaged, exocrine pancreatic insufficiency (EPI) may develop where the pancreas is no longer able to produce enzymes to adequately digest fats, leading to greasy stools (steatorrhea).

Additionally, the endocrine function of producing insulin may be impaired, leading to diabetes.

Diagnosis of chronic pancreatitis is difficult as taking a biopsy runs the risk of causing more injury to the pancreas. Endoscopic ultrasound offers a closer look at the pancreas to identify findings consistent with the diagnosis. Assessing how well the pancreas works can also be cumbersome. Tests to measure pancreatic juices using certain hormones are not commonly done, but instead measurement of pancreatic enzymes or fat content of stools determine whether the pancreas is functioning normally.

Treatment is focused on preventing further injury to the pancreas by avoiding NSAIDs, smoking, and alcohol, and managing enzyme deficiencies by replacing pancreatic enzymes is often necessary. For pain control, an endoscopic ultrasound-guided nerve block or neurolysis may be performed to halt the pain signals from the pancreas back to the brain. Attempts at removing pancreatic stones can be challenging and may not result in much relief. If the pancreatic duct is dilated, one surgical option would be to connect the intestine to the pancreas in a pancreatic jejunostomy to allow the pancreas to drain into the intestine, although many patients still do not get long-term pain relief.

PANCREATIC CANCER

Pancreatic cancer is one of the most feared cancers due to its poor prognosis. As pancreatic cancer lacks symptoms in the early stages, a diagnosis is often made late. Most pancreatic tumors are ductal adenocarcinomas and are typically located in the head of the pancreas where the bile duct runs. As a result, some patients develop "painless jaundice" when the bile duct becomes obstructed by a tumor. Other pancreatic tumors are diagnosed after they are much more advanced or have metastasized. Symptoms that may suggest pancreatic cancer include abdominal pain and unintentional weight loss. At times, local extension of the tumor in the duodenum can cause obstruction.

Diagnosis can often be made on imaging alone. Endoscopic ultrasound is performed as a next step to confirm the diagnosis by obtaining a

As pancreatic cancer lacks symptoms in the early stage, a diagnosis is often made late.

tissue biopsy using a needle passed across the gut wall into the tumor. Cancer staging depends on the tumor's size, extension into lymph nodes or beyond, and involvement of key blood vessels that may limit surgical options.

Treatment for cancer limited to the head of the pancreas can be a surgery known as Whipple procedure. This is when the head of the pancreas, part of the bile duct and gallbladder, and a portion of the duodenum are removed.

For tumors in the distal body or tail of the pancreas, a distal pancreatectomy may be performed. Neoadjuvant or adjuvant chemotherapy given before or after surgery, respectively, is also often part of the treatment plan. To treat jaundice from tumor obstruction, an ERCP can be performed to enter the bile duct and place a stent to restore bile flow.

PANCREATIC CYSTS

Pancreatic cystic lesions are common and often found incidentally on imaging. There are multiple types of pancreatic cysts, most commonly serous cystadenomas, mucinous cystic neoplasms (MCN), intraductal papillary mucinous neoplasms (IPMN), and solid pseudopapillary tumors (SPT). Age and sex can determine type of cyst, and where they tend to be in the pancreas. Of the cystic lesions, MCN, IPMN, and SPTs have malignant potential and require regular surveillance.

Diagnosis is made via a CT scan that provides information about the size and shape of the cyst.

Treatment is typically surgical removal.

• SURGICAL BREAKTHROUGH •

In 1935, during a surgical demonstration for a gastric ulcer, Dr. Allen Whipple discovered his patient had pancreatic cancer instead. Quick-thinking Whipple improvised, performing an operation now known as a pancreaticoduodenectomy or Whipple procedure, so called in honor of this pioneering surgeon.

Gallbladder

GALLSTONE DISEASE

Gallstone disease is very common. In the US, an estimated 20 million Americans have gallstones, and 300,000 cholecystectomies (gallbladder removals) are performed every year. In the UK, 1 in every 10 adults has gallstones, according to the NHS.

There are two main types of gallstones: cholesterol stones and pigmented stones. In the US and Europe, cholesterol stones are more common and formed from a combination of the altered composition of bile, gallbladder function, and how the intestine functions in terms of cholesterol absorption and gut hormone signaling. Pigmented stones, which are either black or brown, can be formed when infection occurs. Risk factors for developing cholesterol gallstones include age, pregnancy, and rapid weight loss.

While most people with gallstones do not experience symptoms, some may develop right upper quadrant pain and other associated symptoms depending on where the stones are located. Some people may experience "biliary colic" where pain develops especially after meals when the gallbladder contracts to emit bile. With inflammation or infection, fever is also a possible symptom. If a stone gets lodged in the cystic duct, it may cause inflammation of the gallbladder (cholecystitis) and infection may develop because the bile is unable to drain. Similarly, if the stone gets lodged in the bile duct (choledocholithiasis), bile may be unable to drain leading to jaundice. If the stagnant bile becomes infected, cholangitis or infection in the bile duct can occur.

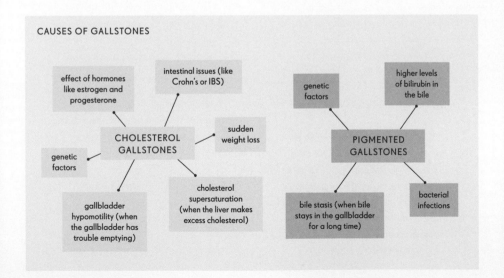

CAUSES OF GALLSTONES

- effect of hormones like estrogen and progesterone
- intestinal issues (like Crohn's or IBS)
- genetic factors
- sudden weight loss
- gallbladder hypomotility (when the gallbladder has trouble emptying)
- cholesterol supersaturation (when the liver makes excess cholesterol)

CHOLESTEROL GALLSTONES

- genetic factors
- higher levels of bilirubin in the bile
- bile stasis (when bile stays in the gallbladder for a long time)
- bacterial infections

PIGMENTED GALLSTONES

Diagnosis through blood tests may help indicate whether there is a blockage in the bile duct or an infection in the gallbladder. Because these stones often do not show up on X-ray, other kinds of scans may be required to help locate the stones.

Treatment of infected bile requires the urgent removal of the offending stone. In cholecystitis, the main method would be to remove the gallbladder, except in patients who are too unstable to undergo surgery in which case a cholecystostomy tube can be placed through the skin to drain the gallbladder of pus.

Because the bile duct can be more difficult to access, the main method of stone retrieval is a procedure called endoscopic retrograde cholangiopancreatography (ERCP) where the bile duct is accessed through the opening where the bile usually drains into the intestine. Sometimes stones can be large and stubborn and require multiple techniques to fragment the stone, using crushing baskets, shock waves, or lasers, before removing the stone in pieces. When possible, the gallbladder should also be removed promptly to prevent recurrence.

Many patients with gallbladder cancer have a history of gallstones.

Methods aimed at "dissolving" stones with a medication called ursodeoxycholic acid (ursodiol) are inconsistent depending on the size of the stone and mainly reserved as a secondary option for those who cannot undergo procedural stone removal.

PRIMARY SCLEROSING CHOLANGITIS (PSC)

Primary sclerosing cholangitis is a condition that causes inflammation and destruction of the bile ducts and affects around 10 per 100,000 people in North America. PSC is closely linked to inflammatory bowel disease, with 90 percent of patients with PSC having IBD (mostly ulcerative colitis). However, only a small fraction of patients with IBD have PSC. The disease progressively worsens where at first there are no symptoms, then there are detectable abnormalities in the blood, then symptoms of jaundice or itchiness occur, before cirrhosis and end-stage liver disease. Cholangiocarcinoma, or bile duct cancer, is also a possible complication.

Diagnosis is made from blood tests, a cholangiogram, which is an imaging technique to view the bile ducts, and, if necessary, a liver biopsy to confirm the diagnosis.

Treatment is focused on managing symptoms and complications as there is no targeted medication to treat PSC. The only treatment with demonstrated benefit is liver transplantation. Median survival for patients with symptoms is about 8 to 9 years.

GALLBLADDER CANCER

Gallbladder cancer is relatively rare in Western countries. Although many patients with gallbladder cancer have a history of gallstones, there is no clear causal association between stones and gallbladder cancer. Besides gallbladder polyps, some anatomic anomalies, and porcelain gallbladder (calcified gallbladder) may be risk factors that require preventative gallbladder removal.

Like gallbladder polyps, gallbladder cancer is often diagnosed incidentally upon gallbladder removal for other reasons. There are a variety of different growths that can occur in the gallbladder, including cholesterol deposits, adenomyomas, inflammatory polyps, and adenomas. Of these, adenomas are the only polyps that are precancerous and require gallbladder removal. However, these polyps are difficult to diagnose because they often do not cause symptoms and are hard to distinguish on imaging alone.

Diagnosis is often made incidentally after the gallbladder is removed for another reason (like gallstone disease).

Treatment is the surgical removal of the gallbladder and/or radiotherapy.

• CANCER OF THE BILE DUCT•

Cholangiocarcinoma has a notoriously poor prognosis. In most cases, the cause is unknown, although certain underlying bile duct cysts, parasites, and toxins have been linked to the cancer. Because the bile duct is a small organ, diagnosis is often difficult and obstructive complications arise quickly. Furthermore, given the nature of cancer, it can be difficult to diagnose even with cholangioscopy-guided biopsy. The only definitive treatment is surgical resection, although the ability to do this is dependent on the location of the cancer

Q: IS IT SAFE TO EAT SEEDS IF I HAVE COLONIC DIVERTICULA, OR WILL I GO ON TO DEVELOP DIVERTICULITIS?

A: There is no increased risk of developing diverticulitis if you choose to eat seeds, nuts, corn, or other foods.

—

Q: IS LEAKY GUT A REAL DIAGNOSIS?

A: Everyone has some degree of intestinal permeability, but "leaky gut" is not a formally recognized diagnosis, or disease itself. There may be increased intestinal permeability with certain conditions like celiac disease or IBD that allow certain things to pass through the intestinal barrier. However, there is no clear scientific basis to cite leaky gut as the sole cause of any specific disease.

—

Q: IS COLORECTAL CANCER CAUSED BY A SEXUALLY TRANSMITTED INFECTION LIKE HPV?

A: While anal cancer may be linked to HPV, colorectal cancer develops following a different pathway altogether and is not associated with any sexually transmitted infection.

—

Q: WHY ARE PEOPLE SCARED OF UNDERGOING A COLONOSCOPY?

A: There are a few misconceptions about it being painful, the bowel prep being inconvenient, or concerns about undergoing a procedure. However, more commonly there is a stigma around anything to do with the anus. Health professionals are accustomed to hearing these concerns and should be able to help allay any fears.

—

Q: ARE ALL NONINVASIVE COLORECTAL CANCER SCREENING TESTS THE SAME?

A: Not all tests predict cancer with the same accuracy. Some screening tests are specific to cancer DNA, whereas others look for traces of blood. However, these tests cannot tell us the location of the cancer (if there is one) or allow us to remove it. At the end of the day, if any of these tests are positive, a follow-up colonoscopy is required anyway.

———

Q: IS IT TRUE MOST PANCREATIC CANCER IS INHERITED?

A: No, most cases are sporadic, meaning they happen by chance and are not inherited. Smoking and certain kinds of pancreatic cysts may increase the risk of developing pancreatic cancer.

———

Q: ARE CROHN'S DISEASE AND ULCERATIVE COLITIS THE ONLY TYPES OF INFLAMMATORY BOWEL DISEASE?

A: No, microscopic colitis is also technically another type of IBD. Lymphocytic colitis and collagenous colitis are two types of microscopic colitis. This condition involves inflammatory cells invading into the colon wall, affecting the colon's ability to absorb water, leading to diarrhea. This can also be diagnosed by obtaining mucosal biopsies on colonoscopy.

———

Q: IS IT SAFE TO TAKE PARACETAMOL IF I HAVE LIVER DISEASE?

A: Small amounts of acetaminophen (paracetamol) are sometimes okay to take with cirrhosis (end-stage liver disease). Keep in mind, some combination medications include acetaminophen, so it is important to account for all sources of the medication. Talk to your doctor if you're unsure.

———

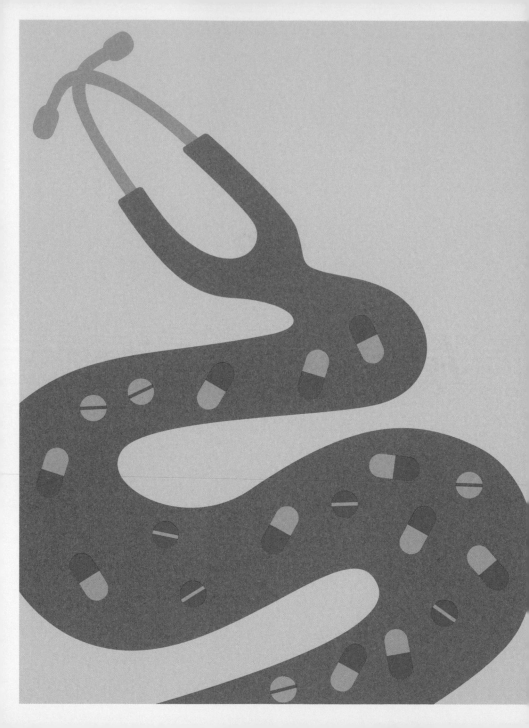

07

At the hospital

getting started

A typical treatment pathway starts with a doctor
who will discuss your symptoms, do an initial
examination, request tests, and make a referral.

A health-care system is complex, and navigating
a hospital and its various departments can be
confusing, even for a doctor. Understanding a
typical journey from diagnosis to treatment and
the roles of different health-care practitioners
can help make the process less intimidating.
This chapter will help you understand what to
expect, who you might encounter, and what
actions and treatment may be necessary.

Your doctor

Unless it's an emergency, you will have to speak
with your primary care physician first who will
ask about the nature of the symptoms you're
experiencing as well as any diagnosed medical
conditions you may have, medications you take,
family history, and other relevant questions
about your social habits and environment.

PATIENT JOURNEY THROUGH DIAGNOSIS

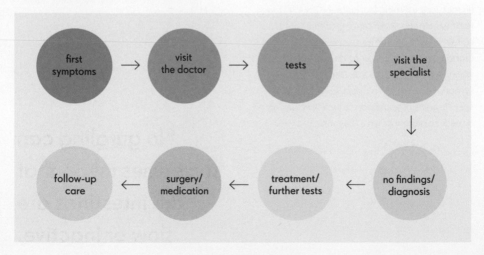

Next, your doctor may perform a physical examination where they look, listen, feel, and perform certain maneuvers to assess and better understand what your potential diagnosis might be. Following this initial examination, your doctor may request tests and, based on the results (or lack of findings), they may choose to refer you to a specialist for further evaluation. If there are multiple specialists involved, your doctor can help liaise with them and synthesize their recommendations. There can be a lot of information to take onboard so having someone to go with you who can remind you to ask questions or who can take notes on your behalf while you listen may be helpful.

Physical examination

In medical school, doctors learn specific techniques to help determine a diagnosis. The physical examination involves looking (inspection), listening (auscultation), and often feeling (palpation) and tapping (percussion) of certain areas. Sometimes the poking and prodding may feel uncomfortable, especially when it is related to the gut. Depending on your symptoms, a doctor may focus on examining specific areas of your body to look for clues of disease to narrow down a diagnosis.

Looking (Inspection)

When looking at a patient, a doctor will often look for abnormalities such as rashes, scars, the shape of the abdomen, pulsations, or unusual skin tone. Keep in mind that gut health isn't confined only to the abdomen. Doctors look at the general appearance of the patient before looking at specific areas. Sometimes skin changes related to gut health are not only around the abdomen but also visible in other areas such as the eyes, as is the case in some autoimmune conditions (see pp134–135).

Listening (Auscultation)

Using a stethoscope, a doctor can listen to the chest and belly. When examining the belly, they can listen for any gurgling (the technical term is borborygmi [pronounced: bawr-buh-rig-mee], which is one of my favorite words!). No gurgling can sometimes mean that the intestines are slow or inactive.

No gurgling can sometimes mean that the intestines are slow or inactive.

Tapping (Percussion)

Your doctor may tap on your belly to assess whether fluid is trapped in the abdomen in a certain area. When there is fluid in the abdominal cavity, as in the case of ascites (see p146), they may use certain techniques to feel for a "fluid wave" where the fluid sloshes back and forth. Similarly, you might be asked to lie on your side to see if the dullness that comes with tapping on fluid-filled areas shifts to another location. They also tap along certain areas to measure the size of an organ like the liver to see if it's abnormally shrunken or enlarged.

Feeling (Palpation)

Feeling the abdomen and applying pressure in different areas can help your doctor determine where the problem is, assess the degree of tenderness (note that tenderness is pain felt when palpated), how soft or firm the abdomen is, whether the organs are the expected shape and size, if there are potential masses in certain areas (although not all masses can be felt), and more.

There are also specific maneuvers to assess whether abdominal pain is coming from deep within or more on the surface (from the abdominal wall muscles themselves). Sometimes they will ask you to inhale or exhale to allow them to bring the organs into specific positions so they can examine them more easily (abdominal organs get pushed down when you inhale because your lungs expand).

The rectal examination

Stigma often leads us to forget that the anus is just another body part like the elbow or eyeball. Rest easy, doctors have seen it all—it doesn't matter whether they're looking at your elbow or your anus—there's no judgment.

Performed by inserting a gloved finger into the anus, this exam can be helpful in determining whether there are masses in the anus or rectum, abnormal prostate findings, anal sphincter abnormalities, or if blood is present upon withdrawal.

It is important to know that there is rarely a single test that tells you whether a specific organ is working or not.

> ### • MEASURING INFLAMMATION •
>
> Made in the liver, C-reactive protein (CRP)
> is a protein found in blood plasma.
> CRP concentration rises in response to
> inflammation. Calprotectin is a protein
> found in poop. With intestinal
> inflammation, calprotectin levels may rise.

Testing

It is important to know that there is rarely a single test that tells you whether a specific organ is working or not. To get a specific diagnosis, your doctors may order laboratory tests such as a blood draw and a urine or stool sample. Blood, stool, and other bodily fluids are collected to test the function of an organ, detect specific infections, or identify underlying genetic disorders. For instance, some blood tests look at electrolytes, blood count, iron level, inflammatory markers (like C-reactive protein, erythrocyte sedimentation rate, fecal calprotectin), tumor markers (like CEA or CA 19-9), and blood cultures to identify any specific bacterial infections. Samples can be taken in clinic or dropped off by the patient. For example, collecting a stool sample can be done at home. Instructions are usually provided on how to collect the stool, which typically involves the following steps:

• Use the labeled plastic tube provided by your doctor, or health-care practitioner.

• To catch the poop, place something over the toilet like a clean empty plastic food container, or put plastic wrap over the pan.

• Inside the lid of the container is a plastic spoon, which you can use to collect a sample.

• Don't overfill the container—aim to fill a third.

• Remember to write your name, date of birth, and collection date on the container.

Imaging

Noninvasive imaging, such as an X-ray, is often the next step in helping to determine a diagnosis. Some imaging studies are better than others to diagnose certain conditions, and depending on what is suspected, a doctor may choose one over another. These may include X-rays, CT or MRI scans, ultrasound, or nuclear imaging studies. Of course, a picture can reveal only so much, meaning a more invasive evaluation may be needed, such as an endoscopy (see p166), which also allows for tissue sampling, surgical planning, or therapy if necessary.

investigations

An endoscopy is a medical procedure that uses
a long, thin tube with a camera inside that allows
a doctor to view inside your body.

Preparation

An endoscopy investigates your upper digestive
system, including your throat, esophagus, and
stomach. This procedure usually requires that
the patient has an empty stomach, which
means a period when no food or drink should
be consumed. For a colonoscopy, patients must
drink a bowel prep to clean out the bowel to
give doctors a clear view of the colon, ensuring a
good examination. To make the procedure as
comfortable as possible, a sedation will be given.
If a case is more complex, requiring the patient
to be fully asleep, they may receive anesthesia
prior to the procedure. Either way, the patient
will need to be accompanied by someone
before being permitted to go home.

Procedure

Whether you find yourself in an endoscopy unit
or an operating theater, the experience may be
unfamiliar and perhaps unsettling. Besides the
gastroenterologist, other people in the room
may include an anesthetist, an endoscopy
nurse, possibly an endoscopy technician, and
trainees or students if at a teaching hospital.
You may be hooked up to various monitors that
display your heart rate, blood pressure, and
oxygen saturation to allow the doctor to safely
perform the procedure and detect any changes.
Often there are shelves or cabinets full of
equipment in the room to allow doctors easy
access to specific tools depending on their
needs during the procedure.

The endoscope is the cornerstone of the
gastroenterologist's toolbox for both diagnosis
and treatment. These scopes allow us to look
inside the gut to help identify conditions

through direct visualization and under ultrasound guidance. These scopes can irrigate water, suction secretions, and insufflate (inflate) the bowel with either air or carbon dioxide to better visualize the gut lining. Most scopes have one or more channels to pass down instruments for tissue sampling or therapy.

Endoscopes differ in length, size, and flexibility. Some have attachments that provide greater access into the bowels, such as a balloon-assisted enteroscope, or have ultrasound capabilities to view beneath the surface of the gut. Ultrasound capabilities allow for needle biopsies of certain tumors and specific therapies that use a variety of instruments. Some endoscopes are used to examine the upper digestive tract and are inserted via the mouth (gastroscopy), while others enter the body via the anus (colonoscopy) to enable the doctor to view the lower digestive tract.

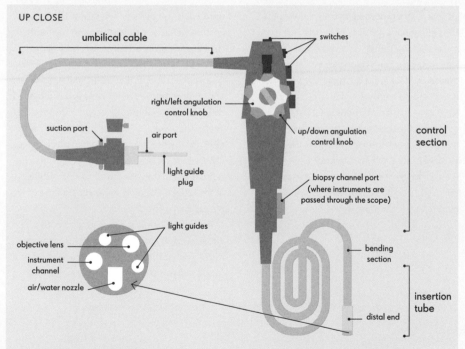

UP CLOSE

umbilical cable

switches

right/left angulation control knob

suction port

air port

up/down angulation control knob

light guide plug

biopsy channel port (where instruments are passed through the scope)

control section

light guides

objective lens

instrument channel

air/water nozzle

bending section

insertion tube

distal end

The endoscope is a flexible camera that comes in different lengths and girths to allow doctors to navigate through the gut, inspect areas of concern, and perform interventions when needed by feeding instruments through the instrumental (biopsy) channel port.

Capsule endoscopy

Getting deep into the bowels can be challenging so an alternative option is using a video capsule endoscopy (or a pill camera) that the patient swallows and eventually excretes via a bowel movement. This procedure can be delivered in a doctor's office.

The patient wears a belt with a recorder that stores data transmitted by the capsule. The camera takes pictures as it travels through the gut, and a doctor manually reviews the video footage on a computer to see if there are relevant findings.

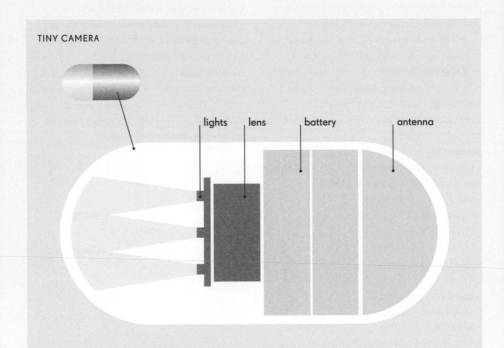

TINY CAMERA

lights lens battery antenna

Compared to the traditional endoscope, the video capsule has some advantages. Measuring approximately 1.06 x 0.43 in (27 x 11 mm) in size, this tiny camera does not require the patient to have sedation as it's pain-free, and it provides color images and helps facilitate early diagnosis. Also, there are pill cameras that have cameras facing both front and back.

Artificial intelligence (AI)

AI technologies were recently introduced into gastroenterology to help doctors detect polyps that might otherwise be missed during a colonoscopy. Health care is on the cusp of a new era of using artificial intelligence to improve health outcomes, and there will likely in the future be many more applications of AI to help with diagnosis, quality, and efficiency.

Only now has adequate computing power been available for artificial intelligence and machine learning to finally find its way into real-life applications in health care. On top of detecting precancerous and malignant (cancerous) lesions, many AI scientists are trying to develop methods of characterizing these lesions further to help doctors with their treatment decisions. Artificial intelligence may one day be able to process patient data from multiple sources (family history, blood work, imaging findings, etc.) to help doctors more efficiently diagnose and treat patients. Even operationally, artificial intelligence might in the future be able to help with workflow efficiency and help clinics and hospitals work in a more organized and efficient way.

Already in other fields like spinal surgery, there are technologies that combine artificial intelligence with robotic surgery to help guide doctors in doing their procedures more precisely and lead to better outcomes.

Manometry

There are various ways to measure the function of the gut, depending on which organs and segments are being examined. One example is esophageal manometry, which measures how well the esophagus squeezes. A pressure-sensitive catheter (thin, flexible tube) is delivered through the nose and directed down the esophagus. The catheter measures muscular and value pressure, which is recorded and the data interpreted by doctors. Another option is a wireless esophageal pH capsule used to help diagnose acid reflux. The capsule is temporarily attached to the wall of the esophagus to measure the pH of fluid that travels from the stomach up into the esophagus.

Health care is on the cusp of a new era of using AI to improve health outcomes.

teamwork

Even among gastroenterologists, there are multiple
subspecialists with specific expertise, who together with
other health-care professionals, help patients get better.

Gastroenterologist

Most gastroenterologists are general
gastroenterologists who have a broad
understanding of all gut conditions and
can treat the most common ailments.
All gastroenterologists undergo training to
perform standard endoscopies. In countries
where there is greater access to specialists,
some gastroenterologists may be able to refer
to more specialized colleagues for more specific
care, especially if there are rare or challenging
situations where conditions don't respond
to conventional therapy or when specific
procedures are required. Let me introduce
you to a few of these specialists.

Specialists

ADVANCED ENDOSCOPY

Specialists in advanced endoscopy or
interventional gastroenterology often undergo
additional training to gain specific procedural
skills to perform more invasive and complex
procedures, often related to the pancreas and
bile duct. Some examples include diagnosing
and sampling pancreatic masses or placing
stents to relieve blockages of the bile duct
caused by pancreatic cancer. Even within a
specialist field, there are sub-subspecialists who
are involved in weight loss procedures, such as
bariatric endoscopy (performed through the
mouth), intragastric balloon placement, or the
creation of a gastric sleeve using an endoscopic
suturing tool. Also, there is "third space
endoscopy" where the doctor can go between
layers of the gut wall to carve out certain
tumors or cut muscles that may be too tight.

IBD

Inflammatory bowel disease is a chronic, complex, autoimmune disorder that is increasingly prevalent. Some gastroenterologists have developed their careers to focus on patients with this disease only. These specialists are not only skilled in treating IBD, but they also understand what to do when there are complications with either disease or treatment and how to care for IBD patients who have undergone surgery. There are emerging treatments for IBD like new "biologics" (medicines derived from natural sources), and these IBD specialists have an understanding of these medications and when to switch to different treatments if the patient is not responding. Many are also involved in clinical trials investigating new treatments.

• REGISTERED DIETITIANS •

Gastroenterologists rely on dietitians to develop dietary plans for a wide range of conditions, using their expertise in nutrition. They provide specific recommendations for certain gut ailments like IBD, or for patients who have undergone surgeries where absorption of nutrients is altered. For patients who rely on parenteral nutrition (food administered via an intravenous line), dietitians must formulate the correct blend to make sure macronutrient and micronutrient needs are met and that electrolytes are kept in balance.

MOTILITY AND FUNCTION

Motility specialists are skilled at interpreting motility studies and delivering treatment for gut movement disorders. At some teaching hospitals, specialists are further differentiated to focus on movement disorders of the upper gastrointestinal tract (including achalasia or gastroparesis), while others focus mainly on lower GI (anorectal disorders). Some gastroenterologists have chosen to focus on functional GI disorders, including IBS or functional dyspepsia, given its rising prevalence and the growing number of treatment options.

PEDIATRIC

The pathway to becoming a pediatric gastroenterologist is different from those who care for adults. Pediatric gastroenterologists undergo a residency in pediatrics (rather than internal medicine) before subspecializing in gastroenterology. There are many conditions (like developmental disorders) that are seen more often in children (see pp75-76), or that manifest differently in childhood. For certain chronic conditions like IBD, a discussion between pediatrics and adult gastroenterology may be necessary to ensure a smooth transition of care. In some rare situations, adult gastroenterologists may be called upon to perform procedures in infants or children as they aren't frequently performed by pediatric gastroenterologists.

HEPATOLOGY (LIVER) AND PANCREATOLOGY (PANCREAS)

Some hepatologists are focused on general liver health and treating conditions like fatty liver disease or hepatitis. Others are focused on managing disease both before and after liver transplantation and are deeply involved in the process of determining transplant candidacy. Some doctors focus on disorders of the pancreas, including acute and chronic pancreatitis and their associated conditions like pancreatic insufficiency.

Beyond the gut

Even when treating a single condition, I often rely on the input of doctors in other fields of medicine. As a gastroenterologist, I'm not able to interpret scans as effectively as a radiologist or come up with end-of-life strategies in the same comprehensive way as a palliative care colleague, nor carry out certain surgeries that surgical associates perform. As diseases of the gut can affect other systems and organs, the expertise of several specialists is sometimes needed. Ideally, all these individuals would meet regularly to discuss patient care plans and agree on a comprehensive plan of action.

Some non-GI doctors help gastroenterologists with the diagnosis of conditions. For example,

pathologists review microscopic samples to help us diagnose disease. Similarly, radiologists interpret X-rays, CT or MRI scans, or nuclear studies we may request to support a diagnosis. Other doctors are involved in helping with the treatment or care of patients, such as oncologists (for cancer), palliative care and pain management (for terminal illness or chronic pain), infectious disease specialists, endocrinologists, or genetics specialists, to name a few.

If there is a procedural intervention that needs to be performed, gastroenterologists will work with doctors who specialize in certain procedures and who will offer an opinion on the risks and benefits of one approach versus another. These doctors may include interventional radiologists or surgeons, depending on what organ is affected, including foregut surgeons, hepatopancreaticobiliary surgeons, transplant surgeons, colorectal surgeons, bariatric surgeons, or trauma surgeons.

Furthermore, doctors comprise only a fraction of the team that is required to support a patient. There are many other health-care members who help bring everything together in the hospital and after discharge keep outpatients healthy. They include endoscopy technicians, IBD nurses, dietitians, physiotherapists, social workers, pharmacists, and administrative staff.

surgery

You may feel uneasy and nervous leading up to a
procedure. Rest assured, your surgeon is well prepared.

Prior to surgery, your surgeon and their team would have spent time behind the scenes planning and strategizing with other doctors to identify the best approach to your problem. For hospitalized patients, this involves close communication between the procedural team and your ward team to ensure the correct equipment and tools are available. Once in the procedural unit, staff will double-check your identity, your medical history, including any allergies you may have, and then hook you up to monitors and place an intravenous line into your arm so the anesthesia team can deliver medications.

There is a wide variety of procedural interventions that can be performed through an endoscope, such as stretching out strictures, or stenting open obstructions from tumors. Other interventions address treating precancerous changes like burning away "dysplastic" changes, as in the case of Barrett's esophagus or clipping a leaking blood vessel (see p162).

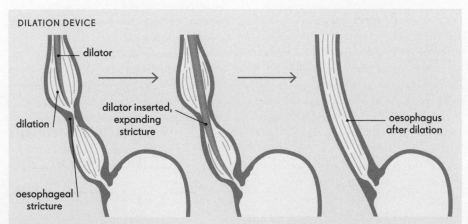

DILATION DEVICE

dilator

dilation

dilator inserted, expanding stricture

oesophagus after dilation

oesophageal stricture

An esophageal dilator can be inserted during a procedure, or even self-administered at home, to stretch out benign esophageal narrowings commonly caused by chronic inflammation and damage from acid reflux.

Going in

Much of the remedial work performed by gastroenterologists is like household plumbing – removing blockages, stopping leaks, and repairing holes! Both benign strictures and cancerous growths can block the bowel and other gut structures like the bile duct. Dilations and stents are standard treatments. Benign strictures can prevent food from passing smoothly through the esophagus, so an attempt would be made to stretch the narrowing using a balloon or a self-administered dilator. Other conditions such as tumors in places like the esophagus or bile duct may require a more robust long-term solution to restore the flow of food or bile. Depending on what the condition is and whether it's a temporary or permanent issue, your surgeon may choose different materials for stents (plastic versus metal). Gallstones that clog the bile duct can sometimes be difficult to remove. After initial attempts at trying to pull stones out, stones may be crushed using certain wire baskets or even fragmented using lasers and shock waves.

There is often more than one way to approach a problem, but some approaches carry more risk than others. On the spectrum of invasive procedures, an endoscopy tends to carry less risk since it enters the body via a "natural orifice" (e.g., mouth or anus), but sometimes an endoscope cannot locate the problem, or reach the diseased tissue, and therefore cannot adequately treat the problem. So surgery may be recommended as the next best step. Surgeons are specifically trained to enter through the skin into the abdomen or chest to treat gastrointestinal conditions. As you may imagine, some surgeries can be very complex and carry a much higher risk than others. As technology has evolved, surgeons have found ways to reduce the invasiveness of procedures and improve their outcomes.

There is often more than one way to approach a problem.

Laprascopy

In contrast to open abdominal surgery, laparoscopic surgery allows surgeons to perform certain surgeries through "keyholes" rather than via a large incision across the entire abdomen. Through one of these keyholes, a camera is inserted (to allow the surgeon to see inside the abdomen), while other holes are used to insert surgical instruments to operate. Since the early 1990s, the laparoscopic approach for cholecystectomy (gallbladder removal) has replaced the open technique.

For patients, smaller scars can often mean less pain and quicker recovery. This also has allowed more patients (like elderly patients) to undergo surgery, when they might not have been as able to tolerate an open surgery. However, not all surgeries can be done through this approach. As you might imagine, some surgeries like a liver transplant require an open surgery so the donor liver can replace the recipient liver.

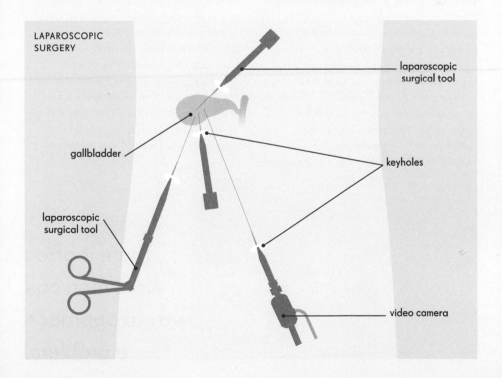

LAPAROSCOPIC SURGERY

laparoscopic surgical tool

gallbladder

keyholes

laparoscopic surgical tool

video camera

Stemming the flow

There are many ways to stop bleeding in the gut (hemostasis). The choice of hemostatic tool often depends on whether the site has focused bleeding or if it's more diffuse bleeding. One common method to stem the flow is using a clip to mechanically clamp a blood vessel. Some clips are shaped like clothes pegs; others are shaped like a bear claw. Another method is injecting medications like adrenaline to constrict the blood vessel and prevent further bleeding.

Cautery is a method to burn and treat bleeding sites, either with direct contact (bipolar electrocautery) or using an electrical current (argon plasma coagulation). Sometimes hemostatic powders can be sprayed onto a bleeding surface like an ulcer bed or oozing tumor to control a bleed. For enlarged vessels in the esophagus, like varices, rubber bands are used to strangulate the vessel (see p127). Sometimes one method is tried, and others are used if the first attempt is unsuccessful.

BEST TOOL FOR THE JOB

For a bleeding vessel, sometimes bipolar electrocautery is used to apply pressure and cauterize the area to seal the vessel shut. Another method is a hemostatic clip that physically clamps the vessel shut. For more diffuse bleeding, a hemostatic powder can be sprayed on.

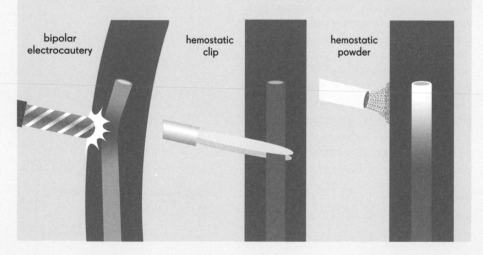

bipolar
electrocautery

hemostatic
clip

hemostatic
powder

Closing up

There are many methods of endoscopic suturing. Current devices on the market attach to an endoscope and pass a needle (attached to a suture) through body tissue to create stitches endoscopically without any external scars. Endoscopic suturing has allowed gastroenterologists to close defects after removing large superficial polyps or tumors, reduce the size of the stomach for weight loss (in bariatric endoscopic procedures), seal holes (perforations), or secure devices like certain stents in place.

Recovering

When coming out of an endoscopic procedure, patients are transferred from the procedure room to the recovery area where nurses monitor them as they wake up from anesthesia. Sometimes patients can feel nauseous, groggy, or experience discomfort. Once awake, the nursing staff will assess whether it is safe for a patient to go home or if there are unresolved issues that require ongoing observation in the hospital. After certain procedures, the surgeon completes a procedure report and provides follow-up instructions, such as staying on a specific diet. For example, patients with esophageal stents require a diet that is soft to avoid the risk of clogging the stent. Some patients may need to take medication for an extended period, like those who need to take

a proton pump inhibitor to help an ulcer heal. Once follow-up instructions are provided and the patient is stable enough to recover at home, patients will need to be accompanied home and monitored by someone overnight.

Some procedures require a follow-up appointment. Any biopsies taken during the procedure must be assessed by a pathologist, so pathology results can take several days. These results may determine the next steps, like whether further surgery is required or when a follow-up procedure may be necessary (like how many years until the next colonoscopy should take place if a precancerous polyp is found and removed). Patients may need to return to the hospital after a few weeks to have certain hardware, such as some stents, removed or replaced.

Some procedures require a follow-up appointment.

cancer

Cancer can affect virtually every organ in the gut,
but not all tumors are the same.

Much of the work carried out in GI is centered around preventing, detecting, and treating many different kinds of cancer. There are different cell types, risk factors, and treatment methods. Rates of some cancers like esophageal cancer are rising due to the increasing prevalence of risk factors like obesity. Conversely, colorectal cancer diagnoses have been decreasing over time, thanks to population-wide screening recommendations. However, rates of colorectal cancer among younger individuals are rising.

Some of the tools used by gastroenterologists can help prevent cancer by helping diagnose and remove precancerous changes or early stage cancers. Other endoscopic tools help us address complications of cancer, especially when tumors cause obstruction. Treating cancer often involves a multidisciplinary effort, including other specialists like oncologists, radiologists, and surgeons. Depending on the size and stage of a cancer, some cancers require removal as well as chemotherapy, radiotheraphy, or other treatments.

Investigation

During an endoscopy, samples can be taken using a forceps attachment to collect portions of tissue from superficial polyps or growths growing in the gut. In tubular organs, such as the bile duct or esophagus, cells are scraped off and later examined in the laboratory for signs of abnormality. Using a needle under endoscopic ultrasound guidance, samples can be taken beneath the surface of organs such as from a mass.

Potentially, an endoscopy can be used to prevent some cancers. Certain precancerous changes can be treated during an endoscopy by burning or freezing away the affected tissue before it turns into cancer using methods like radiofrequency ablation or cryotherapy (extreme cold). Other precancerous polyps in the colon can be removed using a lassolike device called a snare. Some early cancers confined to the most superficial layers of the gut wall in the esophagus, stomach, and colon can be removed endoscopically.

TREATING PRECANCEROUS CHANGES

Radiofrequency ablation (removal of tissue) is the main method of treating precancerous or "dysplastic" changes in Barrett's esophagus to prevent esophageal cancer. By burning away these areas, new healthy cells can grow back in their place.

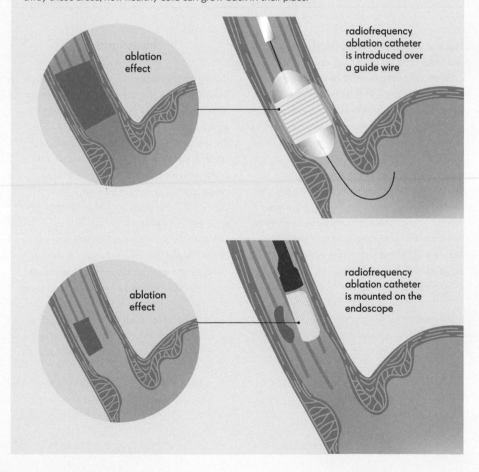

ablation effect

radiofrequency ablation catheter is introduced over a guide wire

ablation effect

radiofrequency ablation catheter is mounted on the endoscope

cancer therapies

Depending on the size and stage of a cancer,
some cancers require removal as well as
chemotherapy, radiotherapy, or other treatments.

Chemotherapy

Chemotherapy describes medications that circulate systemically through the bloodstream delivered intravenously (through the vein) or as an oral medication. Chemotherapy is often delivered in cycles with periods of rest in between. Some of these medications have notorious side effects, including hair loss, nausea, vomiting, mouth sores, and/or diarrhea or constipation. Potentially, chemotherapy can damage other organs like kidneys or nerves and is also considered immunosuppressing, which can predispose patients to get other infections.

However, it is generally accepted that the benefits outweigh the risks and side effects.

Depending on the type of cancer diagnosed, different chemotherapy regimes may be recommended under the guidance of an oncologist. Before surgical removal of a tumor, some patients may require neoadjuvant chemotherapy or radiotherapy used to shrink a tumor in size, while others postsurgery, may require adjuvant chemotherapy to suppress the potential formation of secondary tumors. Sometimes surgery is not an option, but chemotherapy or radiotherapy may still help prolong life.

Sometimes surgery is not an option, but chemotherapy or radiotherapy may still help prolong life.

Immune therapy

For some cancers, immune therapies have been created as treatment options, with many still in development. Unlike chemotherapy, these medications target cancer cells by supercharging the body's own immune system to fight the disease. As a result, there tend to be fewer side effects, as healthy cells (and organs) are not affected. Several factors, including the location and stage of the cancer, the effectiveness of the therapy, and potential side effects, determine whether an immune therapy is considered. Sometimes these medications may be used prior to undertaking other more invasive treatments. Some immune therapies are so effective they have radically transformed how we treat certain cancers, and have given many patients a second chance at life.

FIVE TYPES OF IMMUNOTHERAPY

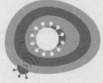

cellular therapy
modifies immune cells to enable them to latch on to and destroy cancer cells.

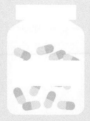

immunomodulators
boost certain parts of the immune system helping it to respond against cancer.

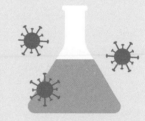

oncolytic virus therapy
uses specially developed viruses that infect cancer cells causing them to die.

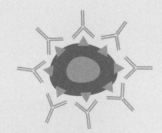

monoclonal antibodies
are synthetic antibodies developed to target specific parts of cancer cells, or to alter the immune system to attack cancer cells.

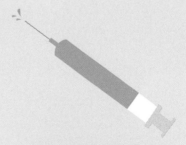

cancer treatment vaccines
guide the immune system to recognize and destroy cancer cells. These vaccines are not used to prevent cancer like the HPV vaccine.

Radiotherapy

Radiotherapy is delivered locally to the tumor site through the skin or through radioactive implants, although there are some radioactive drugs that circulate systemically throughout the body. Radiotherapy acts by damaging the DNA of the cancer cell. Side effects of radiotherapy also vary but can range from fatigue, skin irritation, and nausea to diarrhea and fertility problems. Some radiotherapy-related changes may not appear until months to years after radiotherapy treatment is given, like rectal bleeding from radiotherapy proctitis (inflammation of the rectum).

Endoscopic submucosal dissection is a technique used by surgeons to remove the cancer in one piece. The cancer is lifted off the deeper layers of the organ affected using special endoscopic knives. If the tumor has invaded too deeply or is too large for endoscopic removal, surgery may be the preferred option. Depending on the location of the cancer, different surgeries may be recommended.

The surgery most often recommended for esophageal cancer is an esophagostomy or removal of part of the esophagus. Similarly for colorectal cancer, portions of the colon may be removed, and how the remainder of the colon is reconnected may vary depending on the location of the tumor.

Treating complications of cancer also falls within the field of gastroenterology, whether it's the indirect effects of a pancreatic tumor pushing against other neighboring structures such as the bile duct, or the gastrointestinal side effects of cancer treatment.

Radiotherapy acts by damaging the DNA of the cancer cell.

over-the-counter gut medications

Serious and/or persistent symptoms require medical
attention, but over-the-counter medications can be
a convenient option for transient problems.

In a pharmacy, you can often find medications for common ailments like heartburn or constipation. Be sure to read the packaging and instructions closely and see your doctor if you find yourself relying on these medications long term to stay comfortable.

HEARTBURN MEDICATION

Antacids are medications that neutralize acid but do not affect acid production. Most antacids include either calcium carbonate, magnesium hydroxide, aluminum hydroxide, or sodium bicarbonate. Some antacids have other effects, for example, magnesium hydroxide acts as a laxative and aluminum hydroxide as a protective barrier to coat the surface of the stomach. Some are found, in combination with other medications, to help with symptoms like gas.

Proton pump inhibitors (PPIs) belong to a class of drugs with names that end in "-prazole" such as omeprazole, used to control acid production in the stomach. PPIs are recommended as a first-line treatment for acid reflux, but this medication is also used to heal stomach ulcers. Often the goal is to limit PPIs to short-term use, but some people depend on PPIs long term to

control symptoms. The evidence so far shows that long-term use can lead to diarrhea, and osteoporosis and bone fractures as stomach acid is involved in the absorption of some nutrients like calcium, magnesium, and vitamin B12. Reduced stomach acid might lead to some gut bacteria multiplying and causing diarrheal illness, too. Links to kidney problems and dementia have not been well demonstrated.

H2 blockers stop the production of histamine, which stimulates cells in the stomach to make acid. H2 blockers end in "-tidine" and several brands available over the counter include famotidine (Pepcid), ranitidine (Zantac), and cimetidine (Tagamet). Generally, H2 blockers are thought to be less effective than PPIs.

Antacids are medications that neutralize acid but do not affect acid production.

LAXATIVES AND STOOL SOFTENERS

Stimulant laxatives stimulate the nerves that cause the muscles of the gut to contract and move stool through the colon. Bisacodyl (Dulcolax) and senna are examples of stimulant laxatives that work through this mechanism. Long-term use of stimulant laxatives may result in desensitization and dependence, where constipation may result if the medication is stopped.

Glycerine suppositories are inserted into the rectum, where the suppository then melts. Because glycerine is a sugar alcohol, it attracts water, which increases the water content of the stool. The glycerine also irritates the lining of the rectum, which stimulates the muscles to contract and push out the stool.

Docusate (Colace) is a stool softener that increases the amount of water in the stool and allows fat and water to penetrate the stool more easily to make it softer. Unlike stimulant laxatives, docusate does not stimulate any muscle activity.

Osmotic laxatives draw fluid into the stool. The scientific phenomenon of osmosis explains how water moves across a membrane from a low water concentration to a high water concentration. Examples of osmotic laxatives include polyethylene glycol (Miralax), lactulose, or magnesium hydroxide.

Fiber supplements can be considered a type of laxative, but they also have bulking properties. Fiber comes in two forms: soluble and insoluble. Both are recommended as part of a regular diet. Soluble fiber dissolves in water and forms a gel, which helps increase moisture in stools. Examples include psyllium husk (Metamucil) or methylcellulose (Citrucel). Insoluble fiber doesn't dissolve in water and can serve to flush out the gut. Examples of this include wheat dextrin (Benefiber) and bran. Soluble fiber is fermented by gut bacteria, while insoluble fiber is undigested.

ANTIDIARRHEALS

Antidiarrheals slow the movement of the intestine. The main over-the-counter antidiarrheal is loperamide (Imodium). Loperamide slows peristalsis. This medication does not cross into the brain, which allows its effects to target the intestines and provide diarrhea relief. Bismuth salicylate also has antidiarrheal properties.

Bismuth salicylate is the active ingredient in over-the-counter medications like Pepto Bismol or Kaopectate. Bismuth salicylate is an antacid, but it can also help relieve nausea, indigestion, and diarrhea by coating the lining of the gut and protect it from further irritation and inflammation. Taking Pepto Bismol may turn your stools black, so don't be alarmed if you notice this!

natural treatments

Natural remedies and complementary therapies can
often provide relief to patients with persistent symptoms.

• NATURAL OR PRESCRIPTION? •

My goal as a doctor is to minimize the use of prescription medications,
and I recognize that conventional medications and procedures are often inadequate.
However, it is important to note that natural remedies are not typically subjected to
the same scientific review processes that medications are, and therefore claims may
not be vetted and any benefit difficult to prove. The term "natural" can mean
different things depending on the product, and while some people may prefer
nonsynthetic options, there are situations where choosing natural remedies
may prove counterproductive. I would always recommend seeking professional
advice to get relief for a specific condition.

Given the gut-brain connection, there may
be natural treatments that can improve
symptoms and disease by acting on this
pathway. Biofeedback therapy, for instance,
is an important and well-established part of
the remedial plan for several GI conditions.
This mind-body training involves using visual
or auditory feedback to control automatic body
functions such as breathing. Depending on the
treatment sought, it may be advisable to seek
professional expertise.

Probiotics

Probiotics are referred to as "good" bacteria that
are ingested either as a supplement or probiotic
fermented food, such as "live" yogurt and milk.
Probiotic supplements are often found in health
food stores that offer a variety of formulations,
including bacteria like *Lactobacillus acidophilus*,
bifidobacterium lactis, Saccharomyces boulardii,
and *Streptococcus thermophilus*. From a
scientific perspective, it remains unclear

which specific bacterial strains should be recommended, which conditions they benefit the most, the differences in quality between different probiotic brands, and at what dosages probiotics should be given and over what time.

According to the latest evidence-based guidelines published by the American Gastroenterological Association, a leading professional society, there are three scenarios where probiotics would be recommended: in adults and children taking antibiotics, patients with an inflammatory disease such as IBD, patients who have had surgery for pouchitis, and preterm, low-birthweight infants where certain bacterial strains of probiotics may help to prevent a life-threatening condition called necrotizing enterocolitis, in which bacterial infection can lead to inflammation of the

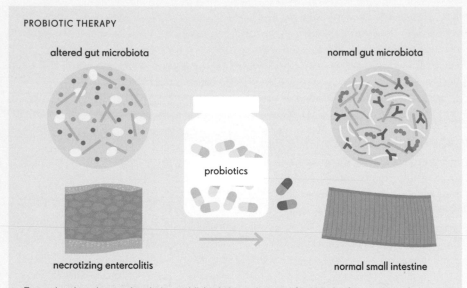

PROBIOTIC THERAPY

altered gut microbiota

normal gut microbiota

probiotics

necrotizing entercolitis

normal small intestine

Every day there is new data being published about the use of probiotics for a variety of conditions. Experts are constantly assessing the adequacy and quality of the evidence to develop recommendations for use of probiotics for specific situations and conditions.

intestine and cell death. If you're interested in trying probiotics it is a good idea to talk to your gastroenterologist or doctor to understand if it is safe to do so and consider starting in small doses to see how your body responds.

Exercise

Physical activity is important not only for heart health but also for boosting circulation and oxygenation of the gut, improving overall function, stimulating bowel movements in patients with constipation, and reducing the risk of cancer. Moreover, exercise can help in stress reduction, which is important when considering the gut-brain axis.

Yoga is a form of physical activity that focuses on both body and mind. Multiple studies have investigated the potential benefits of yoga and other similar exercises in reducing stimulation and stressors that could worsen conditions involving the gut-brain axis such as IBS. Research is also ongoing to assess the effects of exercise on the gut microbiota.

Therapy

Behavioral therapy can be helpful for conditions traditionally associated with the gut-brain axis, and also for other conditions such as pelvic floor dyssynergia. Some psychological interventions like cognitive behavioral therapy (CBT) and hypnotherapy may provide benefits for patients with IBS. Pelvic floor therapy with biofeedback educates patients on how specific muscles act during defecation, and the importance of training disordered muscle coordination when using the toilet. Behavioral therapy could play an important role in reducing anxiety around various gastrointestinal conditions and in supporting patients to cope with chronic symptoms like pain or nausea.

Exercise can help in stress reduction, which is important when considering the gut-brain axis

Herbs and spices

Herbs are commonly used for GI ailments. Anecdotally, ginger and ginger teas have been used as traditional remedies for nausea and vomiting. Evidence has shown the benefits of over-the-counter peppermint oil formulations in patients with IBS, helping relax intestinal muscles. Curcumin, the active ingredient of turmeric, has also been studied for its anti-inflammatory properties and its potential application in conditions like inflammatory bowel disease.

Cannabis

Cannabis can be legally obtained or prescribed for medical use in some countries or regions. It has been found to provide symptomatic relief for certain conditions like IBD.

However, prolonged use of cannabis may worsen some symptoms and lead to conditions like cannabinoid hyperemesis syndrome, where patients may experience severe recurrent vomiting.

Acupuncture

Acupuncture is a traditional therapy where thin needles are inserted through the skin at various points. It has long been used in traditional Chinese medicine (TCM) to alleviate gastrointestinal symptoms. While there is no consensus on the efficacy of acupuncture for specific conditions or the exact mechanism of the therapy, some of the proposed benefits include improving gut motility, gut barrier integrity, and sensitivity, although more research is needed.

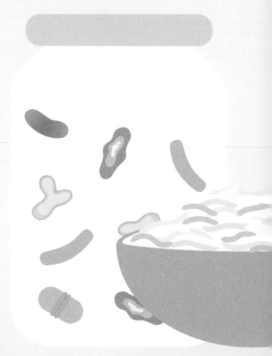

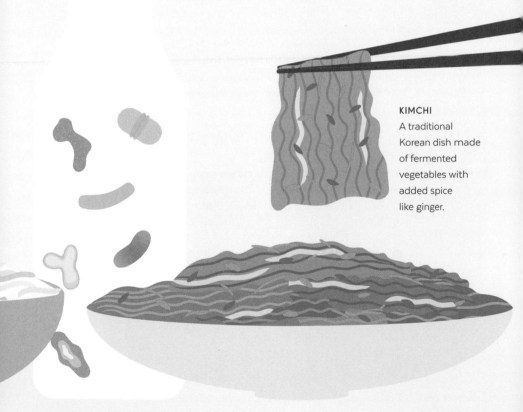

• FERMENTED FOODS •

Considered beneficial for digestion and health, traditional fermented foods include sauerkraut, kimchi, kombucha, and kefir. These foods are made by adding live microorganisms, like bacteria or yeast. Not all fermented foods contain probiotics.

KIMCHI
A traditional Korean dish made of fermented vegetables with added spice like ginger.

Q: WHY DOES IT TAKE LONGER TO RECOVER FROM SOME SURGERIES THAN OTHERS?

A: Depending on how invasive a procedure is, there are often differences in recovery time. The severity of the underlying condition that required the surgery can impact recovery as well as any other underlying medical condition, which can potentially affect healing time, too.

—

Q: WHY CAN'T EVERYONE BE SCREENED EVERY YEAR FOR CANCER AND OTHER DISEASES?

A: Screening recommendations for each country depends largely on how effective the screening method is in preventing a disease and what available resources there are. Health care is a limited resource and needs to be used wisely; otherwise, there may not be enough available scanners for people who present with symptoms and a known disease.

—

Q: ARE DOCTORS PAID EXTRA FOR USING SPECIFIC MEDICATIONS?

A: Kickbacks for prescribing medications are illegal. Today, the relationship between doctors and pharmaceutical companies is heavily regulated and in some countries publicly reported.

—

Q: WHY DOES CHEMOTHERAPY CAUSE HAIR LOSS?

A: Not all chemotherapy causes hair to fall out. Hair cells are fast growing, and some chemotherapy targets rapidly growing cells, so hair can be affected during treatment. Hair grows back after chemotherapy is completed.

—

Q: IN THE HOSPITAL, WHY AM I ASKED THE SAME QUESTIONS OVER AND OVER?

A: Patients are often asked the same questions because different doctors and staff want to hear a firsthand account of the story. Sometimes things can get lost in translation when solely relying on a patient chart, so please be patient while we confirm that the information we are working with is accurate!

—

Q: MY DOCTOR DIDN'T PRESCRIBE ME ANYTHING— ARE THEY DOING THEIR JOB PROPERLY?

A: Many doctors actively avoid prescribing unnecessary medications and proactively aim to minimize the number of medications taken. Understanding how some conditions will naturally resolve on their own without medication helps doctors decide whether taking medication is appropriate. Too many medications can also increase the risk of additional side effects and drug interactions.

—

Q: I FEEL ALONE WITH MY DISEASE. WHAT CAN I DO?

A: With the internet and social media, you are far more likely to find someone who has gone through a similar situation as you. There are lots of patient-led organizations and support groups that many of my patients have found very useful not only in helping them cope with their condition but also for advocating for greater awareness of a condition and action to treat it.

—

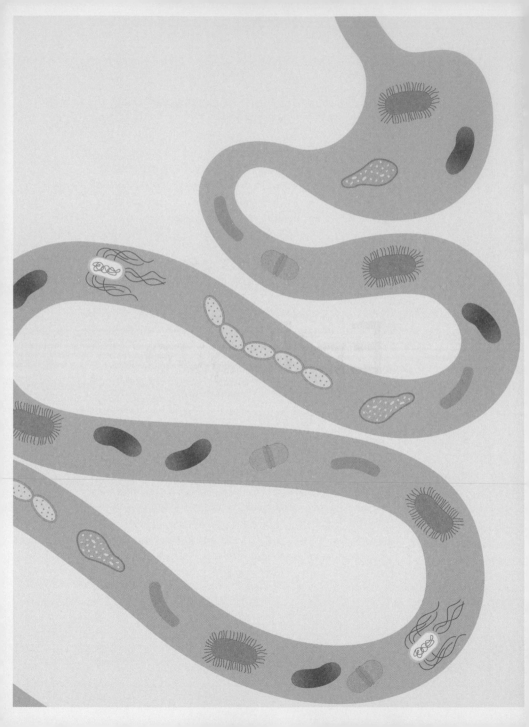

Epilogue

epilogue

Gut health is relevant to all of us. Every day we nourish our gut, we excrete waste, and we all at some point experience nausea, abdominal pain, diarrhea, and other symptoms when things go wrong. These concerns can range from innocuous tummy aches to some of the most feared conditions, like pancreatic cancer. Despite this shared experience around gut health, there are often many misconceptions that lead us to oversimplify this very complex system of multiple organs. Technically speaking, we even get this wrong in our professional lingo. For example, "gastroenterology" as a medical specialty references only two organs: "gastro-" for stomach and "entero-" for intestines. Truth is, our bodies rely on the interaction between all organs in the gut to carry out a multitude of functions, some of which affect our health in ways far beyond the stomach or intestines. Part of what makes gastrointestinal health so exciting is that there are constantly new discoveries in gut physiology and new innovations being developed to treat conditions when things go wrong. Looking at the timeline of gut health, it's apparent how much our understanding of the gut has advanced in such a short amount of time. Navigating gut health can be a challenge when the landscape is so dynamic. Not all aspects of research and understanding are advancing at the same pace. The quantity and quality of evidence have led to recommendations that guide the practice of medicine. The benefits of colorectal cancer screening, for instance, are well established. Removal of bile duct stones through an ERCP procedure can be reliably performed.

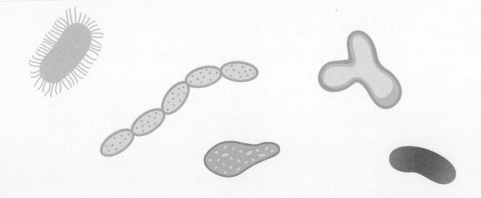

Our understanding of other areas in gut health, like the gut-brain axis and the gut microbiota, are still evolving and could be advanced further with the potential to revolutionize treatments moving forward.

As science advances and we continue to learn more about gut health, the practice of medicine will inevitably become more sophisticated. No single blood test, imaging study, or procedure can tell you how healthy your gut is as a whole. Even when limited to a single organ, we rely on numerous methods to detect abnormalities and establish diagnoses.

Sometimes social context and technological advances outside of medicine have also shaped the trajectory of health care and medicine. Attention toward health equity will change our understanding of gut health for specific groups, and increased computing power has given rise to artificial intelligence capabilities that will aid practitioners in their clinical decision-making and efficiency. However, improved technology

has also shed light on newer concerns around the intersection of health care and technology, such as how much gut health misinformation is on social media. An issue like this transforms how we approach public health-care efforts and introduces additional challenges to how we deliver good care. I view this book as part of the effort to democratize good health information (to the best of our current knowledge) without the distractions of internet fabrications or the stigma of being judged for talking about your gut.

Approaching your own health takes guts. Allow this text to empower you to better communicate about your gut with your doctor, your family, and your friends, and to better care for your gut health. By spreading the word and sharing your own experiences with others, you may not only find some helpful insights, but you will also play a vital role in normalizing the conversation around gut health in the long run.

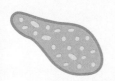

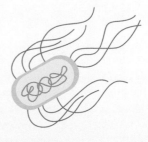

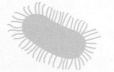

sources

Chapter 1 / What's your gut for?
21 Valdes, A. M., Walter, J., Segal, E., and Spector T. D. (2018). Role of the gut microbiota in nutrition and health. BMJ, 361 :k2179 doi:10.1136/bmj.k2179

24 Mishra, S. P., Wang, B., Jain, S., Ding, J., Rejeski, J., Furdui, C. M., Kitzman, D. W., Taraphder, S., Brechot, C., Kumar, A., and Yadav, H. (2023). A mechanism by which gut microbiota elevates permeability and inflammation in obese/diabetic mice and human gut. Gut. doi:https://doi.org/10.1136/gutjnl-2022-327365. • Margolis, K.G., Cryan, J.F. and Mayer, E.A. (2021). The Microbiota-Gut-Brain Axis: From Motility to Mood. Gastroenterology, 160(5). doi:https://doi.org/10.1053/j.gastro.2020.10.066.

25 Keefer, L., Ballou, S. K., Drossman, D. A., Ringstrom, G., Elsenbruch, S., and Ljótsson, B. (2022). A Rome Working Team Report on Brain-Gut Behavior Therapies for Disorders of Gut-Brain Interaction. Gastroenterology, 162(1), pp.300–315. doi:https://doi.org/10.1053/j.gastro.2021.09.015.

26 Ahlman, H. and Nilsson, O. (2001). The gut as the largest endocrine organ in the body. Annals of Oncology, 12(suppl 2), pp.S63–S68. doi:https://doi.org/10.1093/annonc/12.suppl_2.s63. • Gribble, F. M. and Reimann, F. (2017). Signalling in the gut endocrine axis. Physiology & Behavior, 176, pp.183–188. doi:https://doi.org/10.1016/j.physbeh.2017.02.039.

27 De Pessemier, B., Grine, L., Debaere, M., Maes, A., Paetzold, B., and Callewaert, C. (2021). Gut–Skin Axis: Current Knowledge of the Interrelationship between Microbial Dysbiosis and Skin Conditions. Microorganisms, 9(2). doi:https://doi.org/10.3390/microorganisms9020353. • www.niddk.nih.gov/health-information/professionals/clinical-tools-patient-management/digestive-diseases/dermatitis-herpetiformis

28 Harkins, P., Burke, E., Swales, C. and Silman, A. (2021). "All disease begins in the gut"—the role of the intestinal microbiome in ankylosing spondylitis. Rheumatology Advances in Practice, 5(3). doi:https://doi.org/10.1093/rap/rkab063. • Soybel, D. I. (2005). Anatomy and Physiology of the Stomach. Surgical Clinics of North America, 85(5), pp.875–894. doi:https://doi.org/10.1016/j.suc.2005.05.009. • Śródka, A. (2003). The Short History of Gastroenterology. Journal of Physiology and Pharmacology, 54(S3), pp.9–21. • Barr, J. (2015). The anatomist Andreas Vesalius at 500 years old. Journal of Vaascular Surgery, 61(5), pp.1370–1374. doi:https://doi.org/10.1016/j.jvs.2014.11.080. • Pariente, N. (2019). A field is born. Nature Research. doi:https://doi.org/10.1038/d42859-019-00006-2.

29 Holmes, K. and Guinn, J. E. (2019). Amyand hernia repair with mesh and appendectomy. Surgical Case Reports, 5(1). doi:https://doi.org/10.1186/s40792-019-0600-2. · Haubrich, W. S. (2001). Kussmaul who pioneered gastroscopy. Gastroenterology, 121(5), p.1038. doi:https://doi.org/10.1016/S0016-5085(01)70030-3. · Haubrich, W. S. (1999). Schindler who pioneered gastroscopy. Gastroenterology, 117(2), p.326. doi:https://doi.org/10.1053/gast.1999.0029900326. · Modlin, I. M. and Kidd, M. (2001). Ernest Starling and the Discovery of Secretin. Journal of Clinical Gastroenterology, 32(3), pp.187–192. doi:https://doi.org/10.1097/00004836-200103000-00001. · www.nobelprize.org/prizes/medicine/1904/summary/ · Modlin, I. M., Kidd, M., Marks, I. N. and Tang, L. H. (1997). The pivotal role of John S. Edkins in the discovery of gastrin. World Journal of Surgery, 21(2), pp.226–234. doi:https://doi.org/10.1007/s002689900221. · Konturek, S. J. (2003). Gastric secretion—from Pavlov's nervism to Popielski's histamine as direct secretagogue of oxyntic glands. Journal of Physiology and Pharmacology, 54 Suppl 3, pp.43–68. Available at: https://pubmed.ncbi.nlm.nih.gov/15075464/ · www.nobelprize.org/prizes/medicine/1988/black/biographical/ · www.nobelprize.org/prizes/medicine/1923/ceremony-speech/

30 Are, C., Dhir, M., and Ravipati, L. (2011). History of pancreaticoduodenectomy: early misconceptions, initial milestones and the pioneers. HPB, 13(6), pp.377–384. doi: https://doi.org/10.1111/j.1477-2574 2011.00305.x. · Yilmaz, S. and Sami Akbulut (2022). In memoriam of Thomas Earl Starzl, the pioneer of liver transplantation. World journal of transplantation, 12(3), pp.55–58. doi:https://doi.org/10.5500/wjt.v12.i3.55. · Campbell, I., Howell, J. D. and Evans, H. (2016). Visceral Vistas: Basil Hirschowitz and the Birth of Fiberoptic Endoscopy. Annals of Internal Medicine, 165(3), pp.214–214. doi:https://doi.org/10.7326/m16-0025. · Reynolds, W. (2001). The First Laparoscopic Cholecystectomy. JSLS : Journal of the Society of Laparoendoscopic Surgeons, 5(1), pp.89–94. Available at: https://www.ncbi.nlm.nih.gov/pmc/articles/PMC3015420/. · www.pubmed.ncbi.nlm.nih.gov/30085577/ · Kweon Ho Kang, Kim, K., Min, B., Jun Haeng Lee, and Kim, J. J. (2011). Endoscopic Submucosal Dissection of Early Gastric Cancer. Gut and Liver, 5(4), pp.418–426. doi:https://doi.org/10.5009/gnl.2011.5.4.418.

31 www.nobelprize.org/prizes/medicine/2005/7693-the-nobel-prize-in-physiology-or-medicine-2005-2005-6/ · www.youtube.com/watch?v=adMfyB-eHoI · www.england.nhs.uk/2021/03/nhs-rolls-out-capsule-cameras-to-test-for-cancer/ · www.fda.gov/news-events/press-announcements/fda-authorizes-marketing-first-device-uses-artificial-intelligence-help-detect-potential-signs-colon · www.uspreventiveservicestaskforce.org/uspstf/announcements/final-recommendation-statement-screening-colorectal-cancer-0

Chapter 2 / Digestion and nutrition

41 www.cdc.gov/nchs/fastats/obesity-overweight.htm · www.cdc.gov/obesity/data/adult.html · www.niddk.nih.gov/health-information/health-statistics/overweight-obesity

43 www.usda.gov/media/blog/2017/05/18/food-allergies-supporting-safety-school-environment · www.https://www.cdc.gov/healthyschools/foodallergies/index.htm · Gupta, R. S., Warren, C. M., Smith, B. M., Jiang, J., Blumenstock, J. A., Davis, M. M., Schleimer, R. P., and Nadeau, K. C. (2019). Prevalence and Severity of Food Allergies Among US Adults. JAMA Network Open, 2(1), p.e185630. doi:https://doi.org/10.1001/jamanetworkopen.2018.5630. · acaai.org/allergies/allergic-conditions/food/pollen-food-allergy-syndrome/ · www.nhs.uk/conditions/food-allergy/

44 Barbaro, M. R., Cremon, C., Stanghellini, V., and Barbara, G. (2018). Recent advances in understanding non-celiac gluten sensitivity. F1000Research, 7, p.1631. doi:https://doi.org/10.12688/f1000research.15849.1.

47 www.hprc-online.org/nutrition/performance-nutrition/macronutrients-101

50 www.uptodate.com/contents/vitamin-and-mineral-deficiencies-in-inflammatory-bowel-disease · Weisshof, R. and Chermesh, I. (2015). Micronutrient deficiencies in inflammatory bowel disease. Current Opinion in Clinical Nutrition and Metabolic Care, 18(6), pp.576–581. doi:https://doi.org/10.1097/mco.0000000000000226. · www.nhs.uk/common-health-questions/food-and-diet/do-i-need-vitamin-supplements/

53 www.openoregon.pressbooks.pub/nutritionscience/chapter/7a-energy-balance-not-simple/

47 www.fda.gov/food/food-additives-petitions/trans-fat

50 www.acog.org/womens-health/faqs/healthy-eating · www.nhs.uk/conditions/vitamins-and-minerals/vitamin-d/

Chapter 3 / Everyday maintenance
58 www.myplate.gov/eat-healthy/what-is-myplate

60 www.fda.gov/food/new-nutrition-facts-label/whats-new-nutrition-facts-label

62 Gao, J., Guo, X., Wei, W., Li, R., Hu, K., Liu, X., Jiang, W., Liu, S., Wang, W., Sun, H., Wu, H., Zhang, Y., Gu, W., Li, Y., Sun, C., and Han, T. (2021). The Association of Fried Meat Consumption With the Gut Microbiota and Fecal Metabolites and Its Impact on Glucose Homoeostasis, Intestinal Endotoxin Levels, and Systemic Inflammation: A Randomized Controlled-Feeding Trial. Diabetes Care, 44(9), pp.1970–1979. doi:https://doi.org/10.2337/dc21-0099. · www.bbc.co.uk/programmes/articles/3t902pqt3C7nGN99hVRFc1y/which-oils-are-best-to-cook-with · Sinha, R., Chow, W. H., Kulldorff, M.,

Denobile, J., Butler, J., Garcia-Closas, M., Weil, R., Hoover, R. N., and Rothman, N. (1999). Well-done, grilled red meat increases the risk of colorectal adenomas. Cancer Research, 59(17), pp.4320–4324. Available at: https://pubmed.ncbi.nlm.nih.gov/10485479/.

63 www.cdc.gov/foodsafety/foods-linked-illness.html

66 Maghari, B. M. and Ardekani, A. M. (2011). Genetically modified foods and social concerns. Avicenna Journal of Medical Biotechnology, 3(3), pp.109–117. Available at: https://pubmed.ncbi.nlm.nih.gov/23408723/ · www.ers.usda.gov/data-products/adoption-of-genetically-engineered-crops-in-the-u-s/recent-trends-in-ge-adoption/ · Bawa, A. S. and Anilakumar, K. R. (2012). Genetically Modified foods: safety, Risks and Public Concerns—a Review. Journal of Food Science and Technology, 50(6), pp.1035–1046. doi:https://doi.org/10.1007/s13197-012-0899-1. · Ghimire, B. K., Yu, C. Y., Kim, W.-R., Moon, H.-S., Lee, J., Kim, S. H. and Chung, I. M. (2023). Assessment of Benefits and Risk of Genetically Modified Plants and Products: Current Controversies and Perspective. Sustainability, 15(2), p.1722. doi:https://doi.org/10.3390/su15021722. · Arsène, M. M. J., Davares, A. K. L., Viktorovna, P. I., Andreevna, S. L., Sarra, S., Khelifi, I., and Serguei͏̈evna, D. M. (2022). The public health issue of antibiotic residues in food and feed: Causes, consequences, and potential solutions. Veterinary World, 15(3), pp.662–671. doi:https://doi.org/10.14202/vetworld.2022.662-671.

67 www.fda.gov/food/food-additives-petitions/questions-and-answers-monosodium-glutamate-msg · Ghimire, B. K., Yu, C. Y., Kim, W.-R., Moon, H.-S., Lee, J., Kim, S. H. and Chung, I. M. (2023). Assessment of Benefits and Risk of Genetically Modified Plants and Products: Current Controversies and Perspective. Sustainability, 15(2), p.1722. doi:https://doi.org/10.3390/su15021722.

69 www.health.harvard.edu/heart-health/nitrates-in-food-and-medicine-whats-the-story

70 www.pennmedicine.org/news/news-releases/2022/december/gut-microbes-can-boost-the-motivation-to-exercise · McCarthy, O., Schmidt, S., Christensen, M. B., Bain, S. C., Nørgaard, K. and Bracken, R. (2022). The endocrine pancreas during exercise in people with and without type 1 diabetes: Beyond the beta-cell. Frontiers in Endocrinology, 13. doi:https://doi.org/10.3389/fendo.2022.981723. · Barrón-Cabrera, E., Soria-Rodríguez, R., Amador-Lara, F. and Martínez-López, E. (2023). Physical Activity Protocols in Non-Alcoholic Fatty Liver Disease Management: A Systematic Review of Randomized Clinical Trials and Animal Models. Healthcare, 11(14), p.1992.

71 Kyu, H. H., Bachman, V. F., Alexander, L. T., Mumford, J. E., Afshin, A., Estep, K., Veerman, J. L., Delwiche, K., Iannarone, M. L., Moyer, M. L., Cercy, K., Vos, T., Murray, C. J. L. and Forouzanfar, M. H. (2016). Physical activity and risk of breast cancer, colon cancer, diabetes, ischemic heart disease, and ischemic stroke events: Systematic review and dose-response meta-analysis for the Global Burden of Disease Study 2013. BMJ, 354, p.i3857. doi:https://doi.org/10.1136/bmj.i3857.

72 Schneider, K. M., Blank, N., Alvarez, Y., Thum, K., Lundgren, P., Litichevskiy, L., Sleeman, M., Bahnsen, K., Kim, J., Kardo, S., Patel, S., Dohnalová, L., Uhr, G. T., Descamps, H. C., Kircher, S., McSween, A. M., Ardabili, A. R., Nemec, K. M., Jimenez, M. T. and Glotfelty, L. G. (2023). The enteric nervous system relays psychological stress to intestinal inflammation. Cell. doi:https://doi.org/10.1016/j.cell.2023.05.001.

74 www.sciencedirect.com/science/article/pii/S0006322323013586#bib6 · www.nature.com/articles/s41380-022-01456-3 · Hantsoo, L. and Zemel, B.S. (2021). Stress gets into the belly: Early life stress and the gut microbiome. Behavioural Brain Research, 414, p.113474. doi:https://doi.org/10.1016/j.bbr.2021.113474.

76 Stewart, C. J., Ajami, N. J., O'Brien, J. L., Hutchinson, D. S., Smith, D. P., Wong, M. C., Ross, M. C., Lloyd, R. E., Doddapaneni, H., Metcalf, G. A., Muzny, D., Gibbs, R. A., Vatanen, T., Huttenhower, C., Xavier, R. J., Rewers, M., Hagopian, W., Toppari, J., Ziegler, Anette-G., and She, J.-X. (2018). Temporal development of the gut microbiome in early childhood from the TEDDY study. Nature, 562(7728), pp.583–588. doi:https://doi.org/10.1038/s41586-018-0617-x. · www.nature.com/articles/s41598-020-72635-x · Calcaterra, V., Rossi, V., Massini, G., Regalbuto, C., Hruby, C., Panelli, S., Bandi, C. and Gianvincenzo Zuccotti (2022). Precocious puberty and microbiota: The role of the sex hormone–gut microbiome axis. Frontiers in Endocrinology, 13. doi:https://doi.org/10.3389/fendo.2022.1000919. · Bernstein, M. T., Graff, L. A., Avery, L., Palatnick, C., Parnerowski, K., and Targownik, L. E. (2014). Gastrointestinal symptoms before and during menses in healthy women. BMC Women's Health, 14, p.14. doi:https://doi.org/10.1186/1472-6874-14-14.

77 Lethaby, A., Duckitt, K., and Farquhar, C. (2013). Non-steroidal anti-inflammatory drugs for heavy menstrual bleeding. Cochrane Database of Systematic Reviews. doi:https://doi.org/10.1002/14651858.cd000400.pub3.

78 Lee, N. M. and Saha, S. (2011). Nausea and Vomiting of Pregnancy. Gastroenterology Clinics of North America, 40(2), pp.309–334. doi:https://doi.org/10.1016/j.gtc.2011.03.009. · Gill, S. K., Maltepe, C. and Koren, G. (2009). The Effect of Heartburn and Acid Reflux on the Severity of Nausea and Vomiting of Pregnancy. Canadian Journal of Gastroenterology, 23(4), pp.270–272. doi:https://doi.org/10.1155/2009/678514. · Gomes, C. F., Sousa, M., Lourenço, I., Martins, D., and Torres, J. (2018). Gastrointestinal diseases during pregnancy: what does the gastroenterologist need to know? Annals of Gastroenterology, 31(4), pp.385–394. doi:https://doi.org/10.20524/aog.2018.0264.

79 www.ncbi.nlm.nih.gov/books/NBK570611/

80 www.healthinaging.org/a-z-topic/nutrition/basic-facts · Nakato, R., Manabe, N., Kamada, T., Matsumoto, H., Shiotani, A., Hata, J., and Haruma, K. (2016). Age-Related Differences in Clinical Characteristics and Esophageal Motility in Patients with Dysphagia. Dysphagia, 32(3), pp.374–382. doi:https://doi.org/10.1007/s00455-016-9763-1.

84 Freeman, H. J. (2010). Reproductive changes associated with celiac disease. World Journal of Gastroenterology, 16(46), p.5810. doi:https://doi.org/10.3748/wjg.v16.i46.5810. · Carini, F., Mazzola, M., Carola Maria Gagliardo, Scaglione, M., Giammanco, M., and Tomasello, G. (2021). Inflammatory bowel disease and infertility: analysis of literature and future perspectives. 92(5), pp.e2021264–e2021264. doi:https://doi.org/10.23750/abm.v92i5.11100.

Chapter 4 / Poo
88 Lee, Y. Y., Erdogan, A., and Rao, S. S. C. (2014). How to assess regional and whole gut transit time with wireless motility capsule. Journal of Neurogastroenterology and Motility, 20(2), pp.265–270. doi:https://doi.org/10.5056/jnm.2014.20.2.265. · Kiela, P. R. and Ghishan, F. K. (2016). Physiology of Intestinal Absorption and Secretion. Best Practice & Research Clinical Gastroenterology, 30(2), pp.145–159. doi:https://doi.org/10.1016/j.bpg.2016.02.007.

89 Rose, C., Parker, A., Jefferson, B., and Cartmell, E. (2015). The Characterization of Feces and Urine: A Review of the Literature to Inform Advanced Treatment Technology. Critical Reviews in Environmental Science and Technology, 45(17), pp.1827–1879. doi:https://doi.org/10.1080/10643389.2014.1000761. · Modi, R. M., Hinton, A., Pinkhas, D., Groce, R., Meyer, M. M., Balasubramanian, G., Levine, E., and Stanich, P. P. (2019). Implementation of a Defecation Posture Modification Device. Journal of Clinical Gastroenterology, 53(3), pp.216–219. doi:https://doi.org/10.1097/mcg.0000000000001143.

93 Lewis, S. J. and Heaton, K. W. (1997). Stool Form Scale as a Useful Guide to Intestinal Transit Time. Scandinavian Journal of Gastroenterology, 32(9), pp.920–924. doi:https://doi.org/10.3109/00365529709011203.

94 Accarino, A., Perez, F., Azpiroz, F., Quiroga, S., and Malagelada, Juan-R. (2008). Intestinal Gas and Bloating: Effect of Prokinetic Stimulation. The American Journal of Gastroenterology, 103(8), pp.2036–2042. doi:https://doi.org/10.1111/j.1572-0241.2008.01866.x.

Chapter 5 / What's bothering you?
104 Katz, P. O., Dunbar, K. B., Schnoll-Sussman, F. H., Greer, K. B., Yadlapati, R., and Spechler, S. J. (2021). ACG clinical guideline for the diagnosis and management of gastroesophageal reflux disease. American Journal of Gastroenterology, doi:https://doi.org/10.14309/ajg.0000000000001538.

Chapter 6 / When things go wrong

126 www.ascopost.com/news/may-2022/rise-of-esophageal-cancer-and-barrett-s-esophagus-rates-in-middle-aged-adults/

129 Salih, B. A. (2009). Helicobacter pylori Infection in Developing Countries: The Burden for How Long? Saudi Journal of Gastroenterology, 15(3), pp.201-207. doi:https://doi.org/10.4103/1319-3767.54743.

130 Sirody, J., Kaji, A. H., Hari, D. M., and Chen, K. T. (2022). Patterns of gastric cancer metastasis in the United States. The American Journal of Surgery. doi:https://doi.org/10.1016/j.amjsurg.2022.01.024.

131 Camilleri, M. (2021). Diagnosis and Treatment of Irritable Bowel Syndrome. JAMA, 325(9), p.865. doi:https://doi.org/10.1001/jama.2020.22532.

135 (Stat appears in pullout quote) & **136** (stat appears in body text) Hefti, M. M., Chessin, D. B., Harpaz, N. H., Steinhagen, R. M., and Ullman, T. A. (2009). Severity of Inflammation as a Predictor of Colectomy in Patients With Chronic Ulcerative Colitis. Diseases of the Colon & Rectum, 52(2), pp.193-197. doi:https://doi.org/10.1007/dcr.0b013e31819ad456.

137 Livingston, E. H., Woodward, W. A., Sarosi, G. A., and Haley, R. W. (2007). Disconnect Between Incidence of Nonperforated and Perforated Appendicitis. Annals of Surgery, 245(6), pp.886-892. doi:https://doi.org/10.1097/01.sla.0000256391.05233.aa.

138 www.cancer.net/cancer-types/colorectal-cancer/statistics · www.cancer.org/cancer/types/colon-rectal-cancer/about/key-statistics.html · Siegel, R. L., Wagle, N. S., Cercek, A., Smith, R. A., and Jemal, A. (2023). Colorectal cancer statistics, 2023. CA: A Cancer Journal for Clinicians, 73(3). doi:https://doi.org/10.3322/caac.21772.

143 www.researchgate.net/figure/Pie-chart-showing-different-types-of-liver-diseases-which-ultimately-lead-the-liver-to_fig1_338206302

145 Seifert, L. L. (2015). Update on hepatitis C: Direct-acting antivirals. World Journal of Hepatology, 7(28), p.2829. doi:https://doi.org/10.4254/wjh.v7.i28.2829.

150 Are, C., Dhir, M., and Ravipati, L. (2011). History of pancreaticoduodenectomy: early misconceptions, initial milestones and the pioneers. HPB, 13(6), pp.377-384. doi:https://doi.org/10.1111/j.1477-2574.2011.00305.x.

151 Everhart, J. E., Khare, M., Hill, M., and Maurer, K. R. (1999). Prevalence and ethnic differences in gallbladder disease in the United States. Gastroenterology, 117(3), pp.632–639. doi:https://doi. org/10.1016/s0016-5085(99)70456-7. · www.ncbi.nlm.nih.gov/books/NBK448145/ · Di Ciaula, A. and Portincasa, P. (2018). Recent advances in understanding and managing cholesterol gallstones. F1000Research, 7(1), p.1529. doi:https://doi.org/10.12688/f1000research.15505.1. · www.ncbi.nlm.nih. gov/books/NBK470440/ · www.nhs.uk/conditions/gallstones/causes/

152 Gochanour, E., Jayasekera, C., and Kowdley, K. (2020). Primary Sclerosing Cholangitis: Epidemiology, Genetics, Diagnosis, and Current Management. Clinical Liver Disease, 15(3), pp.125–128. doi:https://doi.org/10.1002/cld.902.

Chapter 7 / At the hospital

182 Su, G. L., Ko, C. W., Bercik, P., Falck-Ytter, Y., Sultan, S., Weizman, A. V. and Morgan, R.L. (2020). AGA Clinical Practice Guidelines on the Role of Probiotics in the Management of Gastrointestinal Disorders. Gastroenterology, 159(2). doi:https://doi.org/10.1053/j.gastro.2020.05.059.

183 Silva, D. (2022). Meditation and yoga for irritable bowel syndrome: study protocol for a randomised clinical trial (MY-IBS study). BMJ Open, 12, p.59604. doi:https://doi.org/10.1136/ bmjopen-2021-059604.

Data clearances
The publisher would like to thank the following for their kind permission to reproduce their Data:
47 Uniformed Services University's Consortium for Health and Military Performance: Macronutrients Chart
81 North American Association of Central Cancer Registries (NAACR): Colorectal Cancer Incident Rates by Age Graph (US, 2012–2016) from Surveillance, Epidemiology, and End Results (SEER) Program, 2019. (Age Specific Colorectal Cancer Chart)
93 © Rome Foundation. All Rights Reserved: Bristol Stool Form Scale (Bristol Stool Chart)
94 CitizenSustainable.com: Average Human Fart Composition - https://citizensustainable.com/ human-farts/. Used with permission (Composition Of An Average Human Fart Chart)
143 Elsevier: Liver Cirrhosis Chart from Optimal control strategies for preventing hepatitis B infection and reducing chronic liver cirrhosis incidence by Mst. Shanta Khatun and Md. Haider Ali Biswas. https://doi.org/10.1016/j.idm.2019.12.006.; Production and hosting by Elsevier B.V. on behalf of KeAi Communications Co., Ltd. (Liver Cirrhosis Chart).
All others © Dorling Kindersley

index

Author's acknowledgments

This book would not have been possible without the contribution of many, both directly and indirectly involved in the process.
To my literary agent, Mark Gottlieb, and everyone at Trident Media Group, thank you for your guidance and support through this journey. I'd like to extend my gratitude to everyone at Dorling Kindersley who have helped me piece this puzzle together. Huge thanks to Lucy Sienkowska, and to Nicola Deschamps (Target Editorial) for both bearing with me and encouraging me on a weekly basis. To Becky Alexander for the initial conversations that led to this incredible experience, and to all the illustrators, proofreaders, sales, and PR professionals behind the scenes for making this a reality.

To my patients, I am eternally grateful. You inspire me to persevere throughout this process. You have served as the greatest teachers through every encounter and procedure I perform. I have met many of you through advocacy groups and online, and I hope this book helps to destigmatize your experience and the struggles you face on a daily basis.

To my colleagues in medicine from around the world who have helped elevate me in my career. To Dr. Christopher Thompson, Dr. Walter Chan, Dr. Jessica Allegretti, Dr. Tom Kowalski, Dr. David Loren, Dr. Alex Schlachterman, Dr. Tamas Gonda, Dr. John Poneros, Dr. Benjamin Lebwohl, and Dr. Anand Kumar for mentoring and encouraging me throughout my medical training. To Dr. Steve Klasko, your support and guidance has changed my life. To Dr. Mark Pochapin, Dr. Fola May, Dr. Hsiu-Po Wang, Dr. Pichamol Jirapinyo, Dr. Allison Schulman, Dr. Kenneth Chang, Dr. Richard Moses, Dr. Jhonatan Bringas, Dr. Eve Slater, Dr. John Pandolfino, Dr. Vivek Kumbhari, Dr. Amrita Sethi, Dr. Nikhil Kumta, Dr. Jennifer Christie, Dr. Uzma Siddiqui, Dr. Manoel Galvao Neto, Dr. Klaus Mergener, Dr. Linda Nguyen, Dr. Neil Nandi, Dr. David Lieberman, Dr. Jesse Ehrenfeld for serving as career sponsors and inspiring me constantly. To the past/present/future fellows I get to work with, you continue to shape me as an educator and I love witnessing your careers unfold. Shoutout to my Brigham GI Bro Squad and my Columbia IM residency pod—you know who you are. Thank you to all the nurses, techs, dietitians, office staff, research coordinators, and others without whom my clinical work would not be possible.

To colleagues at Medtronic, especially Giovanni Di Napoli, for being the most supportive leader and giving me the opportunity of a lifetime. Special shoutout to Kevin Berliner, Kaitlyn Aldinger, Genevieve O'Meara, Grace George, Kate Herdina, Erica Ledesma, Andrew Namanny, Sabrina Zimring, and Sean Stapleton for your suggestions and pep talks. Thanks to the Endoscopy leadership team and to the enterprise leadership team, including Geoff Martha, Dr. Laura Mauri, and Torod Neptune for embracing an innovative approach to my role. To my parents for supporting me in so many ways over the years, making every investment and sacrifice imaginable to enrich my life and instill the ethos needed to see my (very extended) medical journey through.

Special shoutout to Dr. Karen Tang for sharing your wisdom as a budding author with me.

To all the friends who supported me during this project: Dr. Joseph Paguio, Miles Devine, Miki Rai, Dr. Colin Yost, Mike Schnepp, Alex Musallam, Dr. Alok Patel, Dr. Sameer Berry, Dr. Jamie Rutland, Dr. Mike Varshavski, Dr. Tiffany Moon, Dr. Andy Tau, Dr. Divya Chalikonda, Dr. Brianna Shinn, Nikki Chopra, Nick Matter, Mysty Chacko, Ariel Altman, Kate Scarlata, Megan Riehl, Dr. Blair Peters, Dr. Chethan Ramprasad, Dr. Howard Lee, Dr. Anita Patel, Dr. Ali Haider, Dr. Mauricio Gonzalez, Dr. Alister Martin, Dr. Adam Goodcoff, Dr. Shuhan He, Dr. Frank Cusimano, Dr. Kishen Godhia, Dr. Garrett Hawley, Dr. Danielle Belardo, Dr. Spencer Nadolsky, Alex Hall, and so many others.

To you, the reader, thank you for being open to learning more about your gut health. I hope you can continue to spread accurate health knowledge with your friends and loved ones.

About the author

Dr. Austin Chiang is the first Chief Medical Officer for the gastrointestinal business of Medtronic, the global leader in health technology. He continues to practice as an interventional gastroenterologist and is an Assistant Professor of Medicine at an academic center in Philadelphia where he serves as the Director of the Endoscopic Weight Loss Program. He completed his undergraduate studies at Duke University before earning his MD at Columbia University. He stayed for Internal Medicine residency at New York Presbyterian Hospital (Columbia University) and completed his GI and bariatric endoscopy fellowships at Brigham and Women's Hospital (Harvard Medical School).

He obtained his MPH from the Harvard TH Chan School of Public Health before completing an advanced endoscopy fellowship at Jefferson Health.

Passionate about empowering patients with accurate medical information online, he is one of the most influential voices in the field of gastroenterology across multiple social media platforms. He was named 2018's Healio Gastroenterology Disruptive Innovator of the Year, The Philadelphia Inquirer's 2019 Influencers of Healthcare Rookie of the Year, and among 2019 Medscape Top 20 Social Media Physicians, and a 2021 GLAAD Media Award Nominee. He spoke at South by Southwest (SXSW) 2021, and his role in social media has been featured by The New York Times, CNBC, and BBC News, he and joined the White House Healthcare Leaders in Social Media Roundtable in 2022.

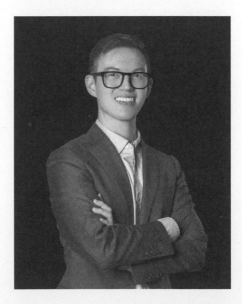

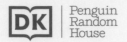

DK | Penguin Random House

Senior Acquisitions Editor Becky Alexander
Editorial Manager Clare Double
Project Editor Lucy Sienkowska
US Senior Editor Jennette ElNaggar
Senior Designer Tania Gomes
Editorial Assistant Charlotte Beauchamp
Design Assistant Izzy Poulson
Production Editor David Almond
Senior Production Controller Stephanie McConnell
Jacket and Sales Material Coordinator Emily Cannings
Art Director Maxine Pedliham
Publishing Director Katie Cowan

Editorial Nicola Deschamps ANutr, MSc, DipNT
Design and Illustration Studio Noel
Jacket Design Hannah Naughton

First American Edition, 2024
Published in the United States by DK Publishing
1745 Broadway, 20th Floor, New York, NY 10019

A catalog record for this book is available
from Library of Congress.
ISBN 978-0-7440-9270-7

Printed and bound in Slovakia

www.dk.com

DISCLAIMER

Neither the publisher nor the author is engaged in
rendering professional advice or services to the individual
reader. The ideas, procedures, and suggestions contained in
this book are not intended as a substitute for consulting
with your physician. All matters regarding your health
require medical supervision. Neither the author nor the
publisher shall be liable or responsible for any loss or
damage allegedly arising from any information or
suggestion in this book.

A NOTE ON GENDER IDENTITIES

DK recognizes all gender identities and acknowledges
that the sex someone was assigned at birth based on
their sexual organs may not align with their own gender
identity. People may self-identify as any gender or no
gender (including, but not limited to, that of a cis or trans
woman, of a cis or trans man, or of a nonbinary person).
As gender language and its use in our society evolves the
scientific and medical communities continue to reassess
their phrasing. Most of the studies referred to in this book
use "women" to describe people whose sex was assigned
as female at birth and "men" to describe people whose sex
was assigned as male at birth.

PUBLISHER'S ACKNOWLEDGMENTS

DK would like to thank Zara Anvari for concept
development, Hannah Naughton for design development,
Sophie Medlin for reviewing the UK edition, Kathryn
Glendenning for proofreading, and Ruth Ellis for creating
the index. The publisher would also like to thank Aditya
Kaytal, Taiyaba Khatoon, and Samrajkumar S. for clearing
data permissions.